FUTURE TRENDS AND CHALLENGES FOR CANCER SERVICES IN ENGLAND

A review of literature and policy

Rebecca Rosen
Alex Smith
Anthony Harrison

King's Fund

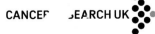
CANCER RESEARCH UK

The Cancer Plan has achieved impressive results since it was published in 2000. However, demographic trends, new treatments, increasing survival rates and reforms in the NHS have altered the context in which cancer services operate. Cancer Research UK commissioned this paper to explore how cancer policy should evolve in response to those changes. Using a literature review and interviews with ten experts on different aspects of cancer, this report aims to stimulate debate about the next steps for cancer services in England.

© King's Fund 2006

First published 2006 by the King's Fund

Charity registration number: 207401

All rights reserved, including the right of reproduction in whole or in part in any form

ISBN 10: 1 85717 549 2
ISBN 13: 978 1 85717 549 3

A catalogue record for this publication is available from the British Library

Available from:

King's Fund
11–13 Cavendish Square
London W1G 0AN
Tel: 020 7307 2591
Fax: 020 7307 2801
Email: publications@kingsfund.org.uk
www.kingsfund.org.uk/publications

Edited by Final Draft Consultancy and Lyn Whitfield
Typeset by Florence Production Ltd, Stoodleigh, Devon
Printed in the UK by Hobbs

This report has been commissioned by Cancer Research UK.
Cancer Research UK is the world's leading independent organisation dedicated to cancer research, with an annual research spend of over £217 million. We support research into all aspects of cancer through the work of more than 3,000 scientists, doctors and nurses.

Contents

List of figures

Acknowledgements

We are very grateful to the ten interviewees who made time in their busy schedules at short notice to talk to us.

Thanks also to Ros West for her administrative support and to Catherine Foot and Hilary Jackson for their involvement and support and to Ruth Thorlby and Richard Lewis for helpful comments on earlier drafts.

Introduction

This report presents an overview of recent cancer policy and argues that the time is right to revisit *The NHS Cancer Plan* (Department of Health 2000a).

The Cancer Plan has achieved impressive results since it was published in 2000. The co-ordination of cancer services has been transformed, with more patients being seen by specialist teams, streamlined clinical pathways in place and faster access to services. Survival rates are increasing and death rates are falling. Further work should now be done to build on these successes. However, there are also a number of gaps in the plan, and areas of incomplete implementation that need to be addressed if further progress is to be made.

In addition, the context in which cancer services operate has changed and will continue to do so:

- demographic and epidemiological trends mean that the proportion of the population living with cancer in remission or with managed relapses is set to increase

- new cancer drugs and other treatments are creating new ways of delivering care. In particular, there will be new opportunities to deliver cancer care outside traditional hospital inpatient facilities

- the policy environment is changing with the introduction to the NHS of Payment by Results, foundation trusts, choice and competition from private sector providers and a new focus on care outside hospitals, as a result of the White Paper, *Our Health, Our Care, Our Say* (Department of Health 2006c).

This report was commissioned from the King's Fund by Cancer Research UK in order to stimulate debate about the next steps for cancer policy in England.

The time is right for such a debate, because NHS structures are starting to change in response to the new policy environment. We have an opportunity to mould these changes to equip cancer services to deal effectively with the challenges they will face in the future, and to deliver a better patient experience.

This report was completed in three months between March and May 2006 and is therefore limited in scope. Certain issues are mentioned but not explored in depth. These include the key issues of funding, workforce development, target-setting and how to measure the impact of policy and treatment.

However, it examines the three themes listed above in detail, because we believe these are the key drivers that will determine the future of cancer policy and cancer services. If we can be clear about their implications, and how we want to shape our response, we will be in a better position to align funding and incentives with them, and to determine the kind of technology and workforce we need.

The report opens with a review of cancer policy since 1995 and then explores some of the epidemiological trends and technical developments that will affect the number of people living with cancer in England and the treatments they are likely to receive. It then presents the results of ten interviews with experts on different aspects of cancer, which we conducted to explore their views about existing services and future trends and to test our emerging ideas. Finally, it briefly discusses some general health policy developments that will impact on cancer, before reviewing the key points of earlier sections and discussing some of their implications.

We have identified key areas of work that will, we believe, clarify what changes are needed and support future policy and service development. The most important of them are:

- to develop baseline knowledge for cancer policy and the strategic development of cancer services

- to prioritise research to support policy and health service development

- to address gaps and weaknesses in the current Cancer Plan, particularly in relation to the balance between prevention and treatment and between treatment and palliative care, and around the introduction of expensive new drugs

- to clarify options for the organisation and functions of cancer networks in a new NHS characterised by choice and competition

- to experiment with and evaluate the benefits and drawbacks of a shift towards community-based cancer services.

The impact of recent NHS reform is gathering pace. It is essential that future cancer policy anticipates the challenges and opportunities of epidemiological and technological change as it does so. We hope this report will stimulate not only discussion but action to ensure this happens.

1 Cancer policy since 1995

The 1995 Calman Hine report (Expert Advisory Group on Cancer to the Chief Medical Officers of England and Wales) called for swift reform of cancer services to bring the mortality and survival rates of cancer patients in England and Wales in line with those in other European countries. The report recommended a new integrated structure for cancer services spanning primary care, cancer units in district hospitals and cancer centres at tertiary level in order to provide a comprehensive service.

The government responded in the 1999 White Paper *Saving Lives: Our healthier nation* (Department of Health 1999), which focused on the four big killers, one of which was cancer. It pledged to reduce the death rate from cancer in people under 75 by at least a fifth (compared with 1996) by 2010, saving 100,000 lives.

The NHS Cancer Plan

The Department of Health (2000a) then published its blueprint for the modernisation of cancer services in *The NHS Cancer Plan*, which painted a worrying picture of a service that had suffered long-term decline and underinvestment, used outdated practices and lacked specialist staff and equipment.

In response, it promised increased capacity, including an expansion of the workforce and higher levels of investment in equipment. It proposed that these extra resources should be deployed in cancer networks, based around specialist cancer centres. Its aims were to save more lives, to ensure that people with cancer received appropriate support and care as well as the best treatments, to tackle inequalities, and to prepare for the future by investing in the cancer workforce and world-class research.

In 2003, the Department of Health published a three-year progress report on the Cancer Plan (Department of Health 2003). Mortality rates had fallen by 10.3 per cent since 1996 – although this could not be attributed to the Cancer Plan itself – and were halfway to meeting the target set for 2010. Cancer networks were being established.

Cancer prevention was being addressed by smoking cessation services and pilot programmes that encouraged people in deprived areas to eat more fruit and vegetables. Breast screening was being extended to older women.

However, there were still many areas that needed improvement: waiting times were still high, national guidance on services and drugs was not being implemented universally, bowel screening needed to be introduced, and patients needed more information about treatment, and services and support at the end of their lives.

In the following year the department published *The NHS Cancer Plan and the New NHS: Providing a patient-centred service* (Department of Health 2004c). It announced new commitments to reduce the gap in cancer mortality between areas of high and low deprivation by reducing smoking rates and improving early detection of cancer. It also decided to implement a national bowel cancer screening programme.

National Audit Office reports

Subsequently, the National Audit Office (NAO) published a series of reports evaluating the progress being made in improving cancer services. The first, *Tackling Cancer in England: Saving more lives* (2004), investigated whether cancer services are saving more lives across England and in relation to other countries.

The report found that, although cancer incidence increased between 1971 and 2000, mortality decreased and survival rates improved (although they did not improve as much for deprived sectors of society as for affluent ones). Progress also varied by type of cancer and by geographical location.

The report also argued that reducing tobacco use can make a major contribution to prevention of cancer and, therefore, that NHS smoking-cessation services should be strengthened. It also recommended a series of other improvements:

■ an implementation timetable should be finalised for the national bowel cancer screening programme

■ more action should be taken to tackle the delay on the part of some patients in England in coming forward for medical advice when they have suspicious symptoms and more guidance given to GPs on referring patients with suspected cancer

■ given the shortage of radiotherapy and radiology staff, hospitals providing these services should compile information on the capacity and demand for services in their area in order to assess local need for extra staff and facilities, and to assess opportunities for service improvement

■ information on service improvements intended to address poor cancer outcomes in particular areas should be made available to local communities using standardised national measures as a basis for prioritising the need for additional resources

■ multidisciplinary team working should have adequate administrative support

■ patients in all areas should have equal access to cancer drugs approved by the (then) National Institute for Clinical Excellence

■ the four national cancer clinical audits should be implemented to allow assessment of whether providers of cancer services deliver the best treatment to all age groups of cancer patients.

The second NAO report (2005a) considered how the patient journey could be improved. It found that cancer patients were generally happy with their experience of GPs, with the speed with which their cancer was diagnosed and with how they were told they had cancer.

The care patients received in hospital had improved since 2000, but supportive and palliative care was still not always adequate. The report therefore recommended that end-of-life care should be improved. Again, there were variations between cancer types and between different parts of the country.

The third NAO report (2005b) looked at the Cancer Plan itself. The NAO concluded that it had driven improvements in cancer services in ways that were likely to contribute to the downward trend in cancer mortality. However, it also argued that more work was still needed. In particular, while cancer networks were found to have driven service improvements, some were not yet fully effective (an issue explored in more detail in Sections 5, 6 and 7).

The report found the Cancer Plan compared well with those being introduced in other countries and with World Health Organization guidelines (WHO 2002) for planning cancer services. However, it also found that a number of issues had not been tackled when it was formulated. It noted the need for estimates of the future cancer burden. It also pointed out that the Cancer Plan had not made any provision for revision in response to developments after its publication, such as the structural and organisational changes that had been announced or implemented since 2000.

The report also suggested that a revised and updated cancer strategy could clarify the role of network management teams and the role of key players within a wider cancer network.

Funding

In terms of funding for the Cancer Plan, the government committed extra resources specifically to cancer services of £280 million in 2001/2 rising to £570 million in 2003/4. However, these were not ring-fenced and concerns were raised that they were not getting to the front line. The House of Commons Science and Technology Committee (2002) noted a lack of arrangements to ensure the money reached intended services.

The government therefore introduced a system to check that spending on cancer was increasing. This found that cumulative spend had, after a slow start, exceeded the target figure by 2003/4 and was, in fact, £639 million.

There has been significant investment in new drugs, additional staff and in equipment (including 72 new pieces of scanning equipment).

The introduction of programme budgeting in 2003 means that cancer spending can be analysed by primary care trust (PCT). Figure 1 below illustrates the amount PCTs spent on cancer compared with other conditions in 2004/5, and Figure 2, the variation in PCTs' cancer spend for 2004/5.

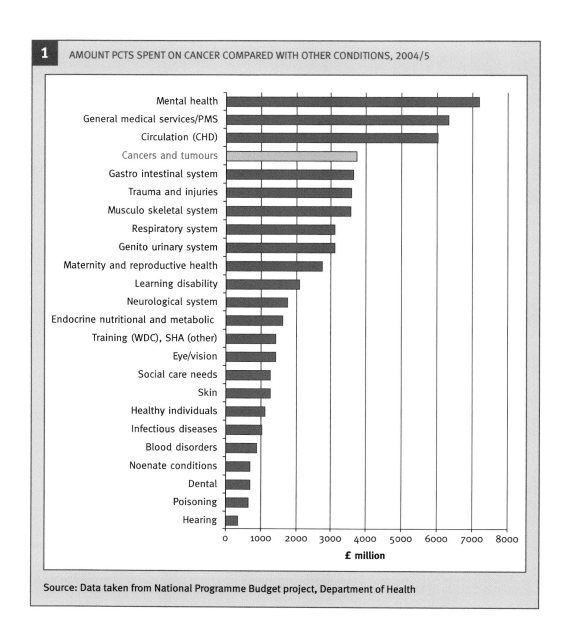

1 AMOUNT PCTS SPENT ON CANCER COMPARED WITH OTHER CONDITIONS, 2004/5

£ million

Source: Data taken from National Programme Budget project, Department of Health

Updating the Cancer Plan

The House of Commons Committee of Public Accounts published its response to the NAO's Progress Report on the Cancer Plan in January 2006. It supported most of the specific recommendations that the NAO had made, particularly the case for updating the Cancer Plan in response to new developments.

In its formal response the government accepted this conclusion 'in principle' (House of Commons Committee of Public Accounts 2006). It did not, however, define what topics such an update should consider or the process to be used to carry out the work involved.

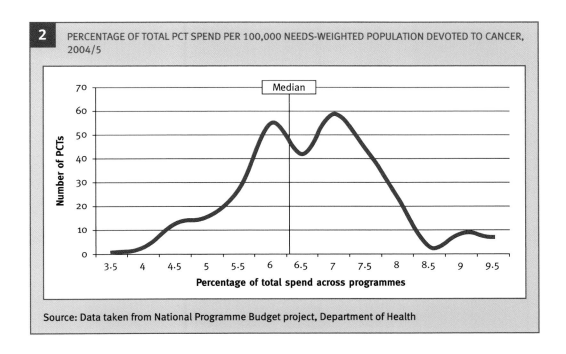

2 PERCENTAGE OF TOTAL PCT SPEND PER 100,000 NEEDS-WEIGHTED POPULATION DEVOTED TO CANCER, 2004/5

Source: Data taken from National Programme Budget project, Department of Health

Summary

The last decade has seen substantial efforts to reduce cancer mortality and morbidity. Early public health initiatives and the NHS Cancer Plan have provided a clear focus for work to prevent cancer and improve cancer services. The National Audit Office has described impressive progress in reducing mortality, improving the patient experience and redesigning services.

But further change is still needed to consolidate recent developments and prepare cancer services for a changing future. In the next sections, we explore how changes in epidemiological trends, medical technology and the wider health policy environment will affect cancer services and we consider the implications of these changes for future cancer policy.

2 The current state of cancer services

A literature review was conducted to assess the current state of cancer services and the epidemiological and technological trends that were likely to impact on the number of people living with cancer and the services they would receive.

Papers were obtained through an electronic search of major research and policy databases to identify review articles, policy documents, government reports and national statistics, and further material was gathered from the reference lists of these papers.

This section outlines recent initiatives to tackle smoking, drinking and obesity, which are strongly associated with certain cancers (a point discussed in more detail in Section 3), and the reach of current screening programmes.

It also outlines progress towards meeting Cancer Plan targets on diagnosis and treatment, and initiatives on palliative care (future developments, including the impact of new drugs, are examined in Section 4). Finally, it outlines the organisational infrastructure for co-ordinating cancer services and the role of cancer networks.

Prevention

Tobacco is recognised as the most important human carcinogen, causing between 25 and 30 per cent of all cancers in developed countries (Peto *et al* 1992). Tobacco control is likely to have a greater impact on reducing cancer incidence and mortality than any other known strategy. Risk reduction begins as soon as an individual stops smoking, an association that is particularly clear for lung cancer (Peto *et al* 2000). The UK's ban on tobacco advertising resulted in an estimated 3 per cent reduction in smoking (ASH 2005), and the forthcoming ban on smoking in public places should further reduce the prevalence of smoking by an estimated 4 per cent (Dalgleish *et al* 2004).

Tobacco taxation policy is a further incentive not to smoke: approximately 80 per cent of the cost of a packet of cigarettes is tax (ASH 2005).

NHS 'stop smoking' services report helping more than 200,000 people to quit for at least four weeks. However, subsequent follow-up at one year reveals a success rate of only 15 per cent (Department of Health 2001b).

Alcohol consumption is another risk factor for a number of cancers, and there is a growing awareness of the links between obesity and certain cancers. Colon, kidney, endometrial and post-menopausal breast cancers are all more common in obese people (Dalgleish *et al* 2004). However, the effectiveness of clinical interventions to detect and reduce alcoholism and obesity are less clear cut than those relating to tobacco, and there is no single, effective intervention that can be implemented nationally.

Increasing fruit and vegetable consumption is, nevertheless, seen as the second most effective strategy for reducing the risk of cancer (Department of Health 2005a), and the government's 'five-a-day' policy directly addresses this. An estimated 2 million children are benefiting from its school fruit and vegetables scheme (Department of Health 2004a).

The public policy debate around food labelling is also pertinent. There is some potential to reduce obesity by raising awareness of food components, although the relative impact of this on cancer incidence is unknown.

Other public health initiatives aimed at reducing cancer have included campaigns about the risks of prolonged sun exposure, regulations to reduce occupational exposure to carcinogenic chemicals (such as asbestos, ionising radiation and benzene) and national screening programmes.

Screening

The United Kingdom has national cervical and breast screening programmes. Bowel cancer screening is being phased in, and an informed choice programme for prostate cancer has been introduced (NHS Cancer Screening Programmes).

The NHS Cervical Screening Programme, introduced in 1988, offers free tests to women aged 25 to 64, every three to five years. It reached 80 per cent of the 14 million women who were eligible for a smear on at least one occasion in the five years before 2004/5 (NHS Health and Social Care Information Centre 2005). In 2004 the overall mortality rate was 2.8/100,000 women, 60 per cent lower than the rate in 1974 (7.5/100,000). If population screening had not been introduced, it is has been estimated that cervical cancer would have killed one in 65 of all British women born since 1950 (up to 6,000 deaths per year). The programme costs £50 million annually (Bosanquet and Sikora 2006) and the estimated cost per life saved is £36,000 (Peto *et al* 2004).

The NHS Breast Screening Programme offers free breast screening every three years for women over 50. It reaches about 1.5 million women per year[1] – 75 per cent of those who receive invitations (NHS Breast Screening Programme 2002). Over 11,690 cases of cancer were diagnosed in 2004/5 (NHS Health and Social Care Information Centre 2006); the NHS Breast Screening Programme estimates that 1,400 lives are saved each year (Advisory Council on Breast Cancer Screening 2006). The programme costs £45.50 per woman screened and the cost of each life saved is about £3,000 (Advisory Council on Breast Cancer Screening 2006). The upper age limit has recently been increased from 64 to 70 years, and two-view mammography has recently been introduced to increase detection rates (Wald *et al* 1995).

From 2006, an NHS Bowel Screening Programme is being introduced in England. This will be targeted at men and women aged 60 to 69. The faecal occult blood test (FOBT) will be used; people will provide stool samples in their own homes and send them off for analysis. Acceptability is known to be limited in some groups. The tests are cheap

(£5 per test) with 2 per cent positive results that trigger a diagnostic colonoscopy costing £127 (Selby *et al* 1993). A randomised controlled trial found good compliance, a reduction in the rate of advanced colorectal cancer at diagnosis and a significant reduction in colorectal cancer mortality in the screening group compared with the control group (Hardcastle *et al* 1996).

Diagnosis and initiation of treatment

Patients who visit their GP with symptoms that suggest cancer must be given an urgent referral to secondary care under the two-week target established by the Cancer Plan. In June 2006, 98.9 per cent of people with suspected cancer were seen by a specialist within the target time (Department of Health 2006b).

The plan also set a target of a maximum one-month wait from diagnosis to first treatment for all cancers, which was meant to be achieved by the end of 2005. Some 99 per cent of patients diagnosed with cancer start treatment within 31 days.

However, recent statistics from the Department of Health show that while patients are being seen quickly in secondary care, they are not necessarily following the cancer referral pathway after contacting their GP. For the third quarter of 2005/6, 47,872 patients were recorded as being treated for cancer. Some 17,114 were referred by their GPs under the two-week wait and 30,758 came via 'other routes' (including consultant-to-consultant referrals, referrals from dentists and referrals from accident and emergency departments). In total, 64 per cent of patients being treated for cancer were not referred by GPs as urgent cases (Department of Health 2006a). This suggests that GPs do not necessarily recognise symptoms as cancer and so do not refer patients urgently.

The third National Audit Office (NAO) report (2005b) (described in Section 1, above) discusses progress against Cancer Plan targets for reducing waits between referral, diagnosis and treatment. For all cancers, almost 90 per cent of patients are waiting a maximum of one month from diagnosis to treatment and 78 per cent are waiting less than two months from referral to starting treatment. The report found that there is still a shortage of magnetic resonance imaging (MRI) and positron emission tomography (PET) scanners despite major investment in facilities during implementation of the Cancer Plan. There is also a shortage of radiographers to treat patients following diagnosis.

Treatment

Of all patients whose cancer is cured, 90 per cent have undergone surgery to remove their tumours. Increasingly, surgeons are aiming for organ conservation as surgical methods become ever more refined; this is particularly the case for breast cancer. At the other extreme, some types of surgery have become more radical; some patients with hepatoma and cirrhosis now have liver transplants. Meanwhile, improvements in peri-operative anaesthesia and intensive care are contributing to reduced mortality after surgery.

Radiotherapy is mainly used to treat tumours with a curative function, but it also has a function in palliative treatment, and this will become increasingly important as the number of people living with a diagnosis of cancer increases (an issue discussed in detail in Section 3).

Currently, more than 95 per cent of radiotherapy is from external linear accelerator (external beam) radiotherapy, which delivers x-rays or high-energy electrons. Alternatively, a source of x-rays can be inserted into an organ in a technique known as brachytherapy (Scottish Executive Health Department 2001) (future developments in radiotherapy and other treatments are discussed in Section 4).

The length of time patients have to wait to receive radiotherapy has not improved as a result of the Cancer Plan. The Royal College of Radiologists found the percentage of patients needing radical radiotherapy seen 'outside a maximum acceptable delay' increased from 32 per cent in 1998 to 72 per cent in 2003 (Ash *et al* 2004). Latest figures suggest we are beginning to see improvements in waiting times for radiotherapy (Summers and Williams 2006).

Chemotherapy and hormonal treatments are generally used alongside surgery and/or radiotherapy. Chemotherapy has the potential to be curative for a number of childhood and some adult cancers, such as leukaemia and lymphomas; otherwise its use is mainly palliative.

The use of cancer drugs, and the amount of money spent on them, is much lower in the United Kingdom than in the rest of Europe and the United States. In 1997, spending on cancer drugs in Britain was ten times less than in the United States and three and a half times less than in France and Germany (Leonard *et al* 1997). Indeed, the United States spends 60 per cent of the global chemotherapy budget on only 4 per cent of the world's population. Treatment in the United States is much more aggressive, and patients who would be treated palliatively in other countries undergo complicated and prolonged treatment (Bosanquet and Sikora 2006).

Other developments

Other recent improvements associated with the Cancer Plan include the recruitment of additional cancer specialists, the development of specialist multidisciplinary teams, investment in additional diagnostic and treatment facilities, National Institute for Health and Clinical Excellence (NICE) guidance on new treatments and additional training for clinical staff.

Palliation and end-of-life care

The NHS has established an End of Life Care Programme that aims to 'improve the quality of care at the end of life for all patients and enable more patients to live and die in the place of their choice' (NHS End of Life Care Programme 2006). It has developed standards for community palliative care in the form of the 'Gold Standards Framework' (Thomas 2005).[2]

Other recent developments in this area include a £3 million per year partnership between the NHS and Macmillan Cancer nurses, and training to develop palliative care skills in community nurses.

3 EXAMPLE OF CANCER NETWORK STRUCTURE, 2003

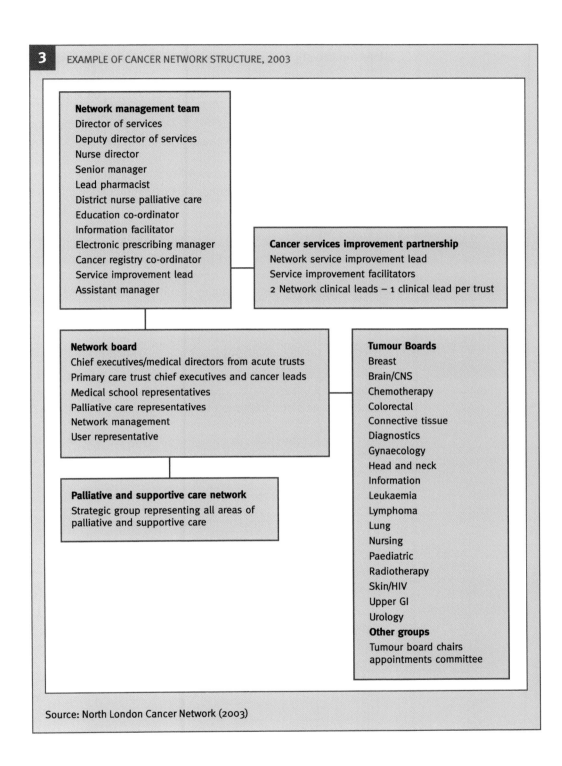

Network management team
Director of services
Deputy director of services
Nurse director
Senior manager
Lead pharmacist
District nurse palliative care
Education co-ordinator
Information facilitator
Electronic prescribing manager
Cancer registry co-ordinator
Service improvement lead
Assistant manager

Cancer services improvement partnership
Network service improvement lead
Service improvement facilitators
2 Network clinical leads – 1 clinical lead per trust

Network board
Chief executives/medical directors from acute trusts
Primary care trust chief executives and cancer leads
Medical school representatives
Palliative care representatives
Network management
User representative

Tumour Boards
Breast
Brain/CNS
Chemotherapy
Colorectal
Connective tissue
Diagnostics
Gynaecology
Head and neck
Information
Leukaemia
Lymphoma
Lung
Nursing
Paediatric
Radiotherapy
Skin/HIV
Upper GI
Urology
Other groups
Tumour board chairs
appointments committee

Palliative and supportive care network
Strategic group representing all areas of
palliative and supportive care

Source: North London Cancer Network (2003)

Organisational infrastructure for co-ordinating cancer services

There are 34 cancer networks in England that form the 'glue' for co-ordinating the many services required by cancer patients. Their roles include strategic planning and achieving clinical integration, promoting cost-effectiveness, improving clinical outcomes and enhancing the patient experience.

Membership includes representatives from acute trusts, primary care trusts (PCTs), and voluntary sector organisations. The success of a network is generally seen to depend on the commitment of its members to developing a collaborative approach to improving cancer services across their area. Involving other stakeholders – including patients, carers, health care professionals, academics and voluntary organisations – is also seen as important.

Figure 3 gives an example of the structure of one particular cancer network (North London Cancer Network 2003). One of the NAO reports discussed above (2005b) (*see* Section 1) suggested that a number of improvements could be made to cancer networks. These include providing sufficient resources to run them effectively. But it warned that wider government reforms of the NHS could strain relationships between network partners.

Summary

The United Kingdom has invested in cancer prevention, faster diagnosis and better treatment. This has resulted in new public health and screening programmes and faster access to diagnosis and treatment for those referred via the cancer referral pathway.

However, there is more to be done. Many patients are still not being referred as urgent cases. There are still delays for diagnosis and some treatments, particularly radiography. And most of our interviewees were critical of palliative care services (a point explored in Section 5).

Meanwhile, although the model of cancer networks and centres advocated by the Cancer Plan has been implemented, there are reservations about their effectiveness.

The next sections look at how epidemiological and technological trends could impact on the incidence and treatment of cancer.

3 Trends in cancer epidemiology

The third of the National Audit Office reports discussed above (NAO 2005b) (*see* Section 1) found that a gap in the Cancer Plan was the lack of any forecasts of the volume of work that cancer services would have to carry out. As a result, it argued it had no clear basis for estimating the scale of resources, both human and physical, that would be needed to implement it. A key element in any such forecast is an estimate of the number of people likely to require treatment and subsequent care and support.

This section summarises published epidemiological data and the views of our interviewees on this subject. It then sets out some key facts bearing on the planning of future cancer services.

Trends in incidence[3]

More than one in three people in England and Wales will develop cancer during their lives, and more than a quarter of the population will die from it. More than 220,000 people are diagnosed with cancer each year in England, and it causes more than 128,000 deaths.

Cancer incidence in England increased by almost one third between 1971 and 2000 (NAO 2004). The total number of new cases of cancer is still increasing by 1.4 per cent per year, mainly as a result of the ageing population, screening and earlier diagnosis.

More than 50 per cent of cancers are diagnosed in people aged 70 or over, and 75 per cent in those aged 60 or over (Office for National Statistics 2005b). Cancers in children aged 14 years and under account for only 0.5 per cent of the total (Department of Health 2004c).

The impact of smoking, alcohol and obesity on the incidence of cancer has already been noted (*see* Section 2). The prevalence of risk factors is known to be higher in areas of socio-economic deprivation. This is reflected in significant geographic and socio-demographic inequalities in the incidence of, and mortality from, a range of cancers, including those of the larynx, lip, mouth, pharynx and lung (Office for National Statistics 2005a). Reducing such inequalities is one of the aims of the Cancer Plan, and the third of the NAO reports discussed in Section 1 says some progress has been made against this target, but further work is needed.

The age-standardised incidence trends for all cancers between 1993 and 2002 remained relatively stable in men (between 406 and 415 per 100,000), and increased by 3 per cent in women. However, these overall trends mask some large changes in types of cancer, as the following figure shows (*see* Figure 4 overleaf).

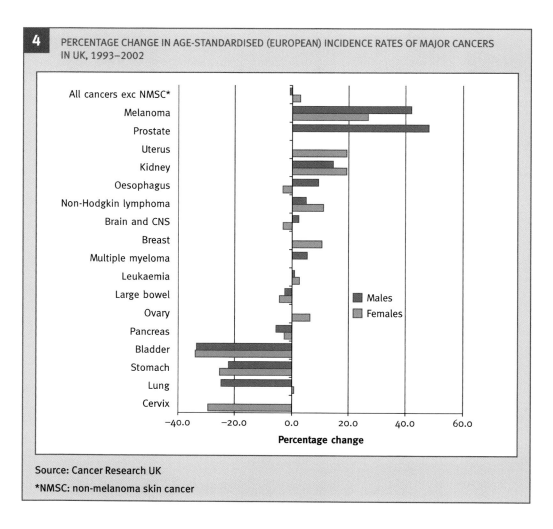

4 PERCENTAGE CHANGE IN AGE-STANDARDISED (EUROPEAN) INCIDENCE RATES OF MAJOR CANCERS IN UK, 1993–2002

Source: Cancer Research UK

*NMSC: non-melanoma skin cancer

Trends in mortality[4]

Although the incidence of cancer is increasing, overall mortality is decreasing. Between 1994 and 2004, the age-standardised mortality rate for all malignancies fell by 14 per cent for men and 10 per cent for women. This general trend also hides large variations for different types of cancer (*see* Figure 5 opposite).

Age-standardised mortality from lung cancer in men has fallen from 77/100,000 in 1994 to 54/100,000 in 2004. In 2004, age-standardised mortality for women from lung cancer was 30/100,000. This rate has remained the same since the mid-1980s.

Rates of mortality from breast cancer have been falling since 1990 despite increases in incidence. The declining mortality is probably due to earlier diagnosis and more effective treatments. In 1994, 14,370 women in the United Kingdom died from breast cancer, and by 2004 deaths had fallen to 12,417.

Comparison between UK and European survival rates

The United Kingdom has lower five-year survival rates for most cancers than comparable European countries. Figure 6 (*see* p 19) shows five-year relative survival rates for the most

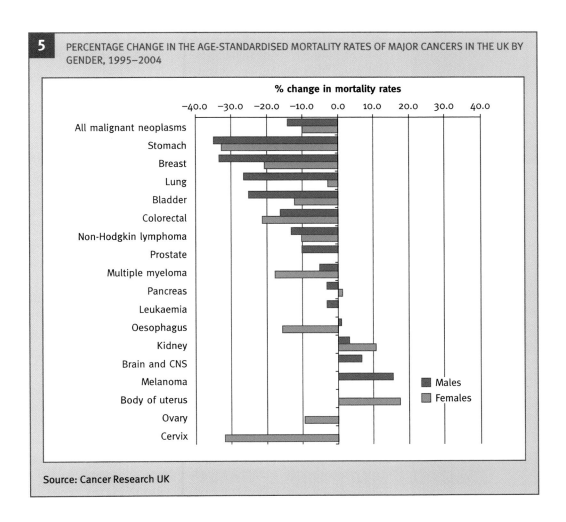

5 PERCENTAGE CHANGE IN THE AGE-STANDARDISED MORTALITY RATES OF MAJOR CANCERS IN THE UK BY GENDER, 1995–2004

Source: Cancer Research UK

commonly diagnosed cancers in the European Union (EU). This pattern is true for patients diagnosed during the periods 1978–85 and 1986–90. The differences between the United Kingdom and the United States are even more stark. Some of these differences are likely to be artefacts, for instance due to disease definitions. Cancer registry procedures vary a lot between countries as to how they record cases and deaths. The registries in some countries cover only small areas and are not representative of the whole country. However, once these variations have been taken into account, it is still true that the differences in survival rates for breast and colon cancer between the United Kingdom and other European countries arise primarily in the first six months after diagnosis. This suggests that the differences in mortality stem from how advanced the disease is at the point of diagnosis and from early access to optimal treatment. It seems that patients in the United Kingdom are more likely to have more advanced disease at diagnosis. However, the United Kingdom does as well on a stage-by-stage basis. There are exceptions, for example, for some gastrointestinal cancers where the United Kingdom was relatively slow to adopt some of the most recent surgical techniques and uses of radiotherapy.

By far the biggest problem is that UK patients have tended to present later than elsewhere. Several factors are bound up in this observation: patients' willingness to present, organisation of services especially in primary care, appointment delays and the time taken to get through the system. Some of this has changed following implementation of the Cancer Plan. A number of these factors might still be influencing more recent survival figures, but delays within the system should have reduced (D Forman, personal communication, 2006).

Trends in survival[5]

Between 1996 and 2001, survival rates for cancer in England improved for most cancers and will probably continue to do so. A higher proportion of women than men survive for at least five years following diagnosis (this is referred to as five-year survival), and the younger a person is when diagnosed, the higher the survival rate.

Survival is the most difficult statistic to predict. While there is considerable optimism in the research community about new therapies, tailored therapies and genetically appropriate therapies (*see* Section 4), many have yet to demonstrate an effect on survival rates. Nevertheless, there has been steady progress in some areas. Figure 6 shows five-year relative survival rates for selected cancers for adults diagnosed during the period 1998–2001 in England.

Five-year breast cancer survival among women diagnosed from 1998 to 2001 was 80 per cent. Five-year survival from colon cancer among men and women was 50 per cent. These five-year survival rates for breast and colon cancers were approximately 2.5 per cent higher than for patients diagnosed during the period 1996–99. Five-year prostate cancer survival for men diagnosed from 1998 to 2001 was 71 per cent. This was around 6 per cent higher than for patients diagnosed from 1996 to 1999. In contrast, lung cancer survival rates have not improved substantially in the past decade. During the period 1998–2001, 6 per cent of men and 7 per cent of women survived for five years following diagnosis.

The future cancer burden

An estimate of the future number of cancer patients is needed to plan the allocation of resources for all phases of care: primary prevention, screening, early diagnosis, treatment and palliative care.

The main elements in such a forecast are:

- changes in incidence (allowing for changes in risk factors)
- demographic change (since incidence is age related)
- estimates of the impact of preventive measures
- estimates of the changes in diagnosis and treatment that will affect the identification of extra cases, the number of survivors needing long-term care and the number cured entirely.

The Cancer Plan did not make a forecast of the number of future cancer patients and it lies outside the scope of this report to do so. However, the people interviewed for this research (*see* Section 5) argued that some broad indications are available.

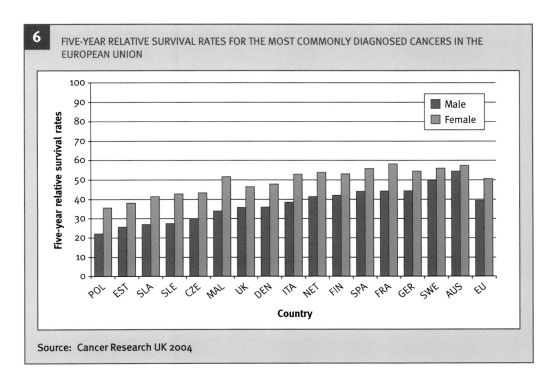

6 FIVE-YEAR RELATIVE SURVIVAL RATES FOR THE MOST COMMONLY DIAGNOSED CANCERS IN THE EUROPEAN UNION

Source: Cancer Research UK 2004

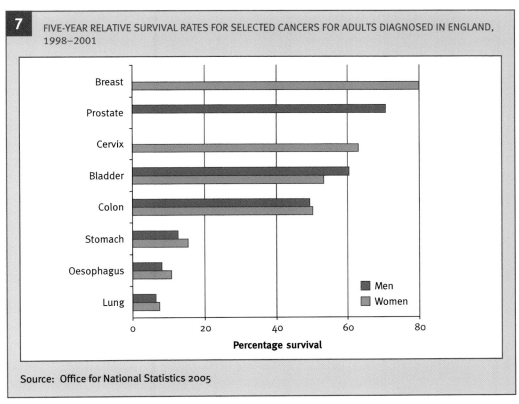

7 FIVE-YEAR RELATIVE SURVIVAL RATES FOR SELECTED CANCERS FOR ADULTS DIAGNOSED IN ENGLAND, 1998–2001

Source: Office for National Statistics 2005

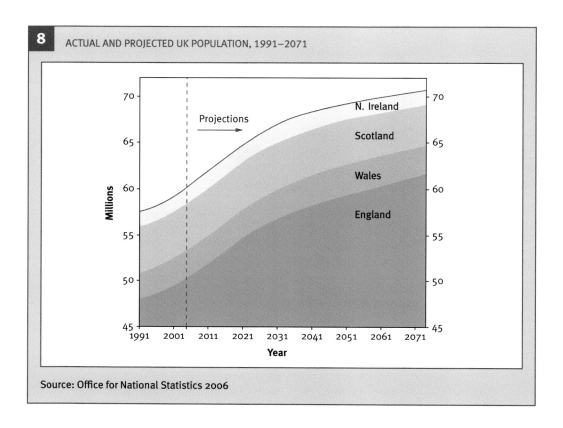

8 ACTUAL AND PROJECTED UK POPULATION, 1991–2071

Source: Office for National Statistics 2006

Figure 8 shows the actual and projected population of the United Kingdom from 1991 to 2071. Figure 9 illustrates the predicted continual increase in cancer incidence to 2010.

The UK population is projected to increase by 7.2 million during the period 2004–31 (Office for National Statistics 2006). There will be more births than deaths, and more immigrants than emigrants. The United Kingdom has an ageing population. The proportion of people aged over 65 is projected to increase from 16 per cent in 2004 to 23 per cent by 2031. This is an inevitable consequence of the age structure of the population alive today, in particular the ageing of the large numbers of people born after the Second World War and during the baby boom of the 1960s.

If we assume that the risk of an individual getting cancer remains the same, there will be a substantial increase in demand for services as a result of the impact of demography alone.

The future pattern of cancer is governed by what is happening in breast, bowel, lung and prostate cancer. The interplay of these cancers is the major driver of overall incidence rates.

Breast cancer profoundly affects the pattern of cancer in women. The conventional wisdom is that rates are increasing in the United Kingdom. However, in the past three to four years, incidence rates have been fairly constant, and the United Kingdom has not experienced the year-on-year increases seen a decade ago, although it is too early to say that the incidence of breast cancer is no longer increasing.

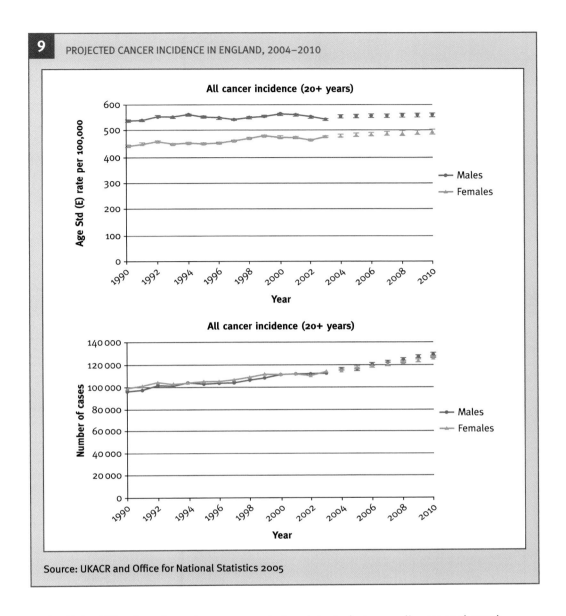

PROJECTED CANCER INCIDENCE IN ENGLAND, 2004–2010

Source: UKACR and Office for National Statistics 2005

In the United Kingdom, breast cancers are being detected at an earlier stage through screening and improved management, so mortality is substantially decreasing. This was evident in the United Kingdom before many other countries.

Bowel cancer in the United Kingdom is more or less constant over time – there has not been much fluctuation in the last decade. The hope is that the impending screening programme (*see* Section 2) will identify cases of bowel cancer at a very early stage and therefore reduce incidence rates. However, this will depend on how long implementation of the screening programme takes and then how long it is before it is taken up by the population.

The incidence and mortality of lung cancer in men is declining rapidly. This has had a substantial impact on age-standardised rates of total cancer burden. It is unclear what will happen for women. Until recently, rates for women have tracked those of men with a

30-year time lag. However, if recent increases in smoking rates in young women continue, this historic pattern may be broken and rates for women may start to increase relative to men.

Prostate-specific antigen (PSA) testing for prostate cancer is becoming increasingly common – although not as a nationally planned screening programme. This is leading to large numbers of men diagnosed with malignant disease, with consequent management problems for the NHS and morbidity problems for men who are diagnosed. There is no clear evidence of PSA testing ultimately improving prognosis and life expectancy for men. The incidence of prostate cancer has been rising rapidly for the past ten years while mortality has remained more or less constant.

As treatment is undeniably getting better there will be an increasing number of cancer survivors.

The Cancer Plan was largely focused on improving care for newly diagnosed patients. It gave less consideration to longer-term survivors living with the disease five or more years after diagnosis. The numbers of these patients will increase disproportionately to the number of newly diagnosed patients because of improved treatments. This will have an impact on social as well as health care services.

Most difficult of all to predict is the impact of policy change, including a focus on prevention or the investment in cancer services made in recent years.

Summary

As the population ages, the burden of illness from cancer will inevitably increase although a dramatic decrease in the number of smokers would have the potential to modify this rise. This will be compounded by parallel reductions in mortality from heart disease, with the inevitable consequence that the proportion of the population living with and dying from cancer will increase (Honore and Lleras Muney 2004).

The increasing cancer burden will drive demand for service expansion, as will new forms of treatment as they become available, with obvious resource implications. The following section describes emerging treatments and the possible impact they will have.

4 Impact of technological development

The trends in cancer prevalence described in the last section are partly predicated on improved survival due to treatment innovations.

Dramatic developments have been predicted in cancer drugs, surgical techniques and locally targeted radiotherapy, although the timescales for these innovations remain unclear. To enthusiasts, they are just around the corner while sceptics note that they have been just around the corner for many years.

Recent media coverage about the anti-breast-cancer drug Herceptin suggests that the benefits from new drugs are now on the near horizon, while the potential contribution of other technologies, such as robotics, remains further away.

Developments in screening and prevention

Although not strictly technological developments, understanding about effective prevention is increasing, as are the options for delivering screening. A cluster of new screening and preventive technologies have been developed that may contribute to reductions in cancer incidence and mortality.

Screening

Trials are currently under way to evaluate the use of CT colonography in older symptomatic patients. It could be an alternative to conventional colonoscopy and equally sensitive to cancer, but potentially safer, cheaper and more acceptable to patients.

The UK Collaborative Trial of Ovarian Cancer Screening (UKCTOCS) is studying 200,000 post-menopausal women (age range 50 to 74) for six years and results will be published in 2012. The cost implications to the NHS of screening and the psychological effects on the women taking part are being investigated.[6]

There is currently no national screening programme for lung cancer in the United Kingdom (National Screening Committee UK 2005), although research is under way in the United States to compare the impact on mortality of spiral CT scans with standard chest x-rays (American Cancer Society 2006). There is also a joint Dutch–Belgian randomised trial of lung cancer screening.[7]

Preventing cancer

Estimates that between 30 and 50 per cent of cancer could be prevented by reduction in risk factors remain extremely challenging (WHO 2003). Current initiatives in relation to smoking, alcohol and obesity were described above (*see* Section 2).

There is also emerging work on other approaches to prevention. Vaccines are under development for selected viral infections that are linked to cancers. Human papilloma virus (HPV) is associated with cervical cancer and a licence has just been granted in the United States for an HPV vaccine. (Cancer Research UK 2006). Epstein–Barr virus causes nasopharyngeal cancer and hepatitis B causes primary liver cancer. Approximately 11 per cent of the global cancer burden can be attributed to infective agents (WHO 2003).

Chronic inflammation is also implicated in the aetiology of cancer: *H pylori* infection is associated with stomach and oesophageal cancers, chronic bronchitis with lung cancer, chronic liver inflammation (caused by hepatitis B or C) with hepatoma. These are long-term mechanisms that offer potential for intervention, either in the form of vaccines or anti-inflammatory treatments (Cox 2 inhibitors, aspirin and non-steroidal anti-inflammatory drugs).

Genetic research also has potential, although the timescale for these developments remains unclear. Opportunities for precisely targeted prevention and treatment will grow, and individuals could know what cancers their genes predispose them to. The average age at diagnosis could decrease as health professionals will know which cancers to screen for, enabling earlier diagnosis, treatment and potential cure. Tailored chemoprevention will be widespread and biomarkers of risk will be identified, motivating people to look after themselves.

New drugs

In the past, the clinical benefits of chemotherapy drugs have typically been balanced by highly toxic side effects. Many are administered intravenously as a hospital inpatient or in a day unit, and additional treatment is often required to manage side effects. In future, more drugs will target tumours at the molecular level and will be given orally, reducing the need for administration in hospital. Oral drugs can be more expensive than intravenous ones, but related drug administration costs are lower. However, the drugs still need to be prescribed and monitored by an oncology team (Scottish Executive Health Department 2001).

Cancers treated by chemotherapy can be divided into three groups. In the first, there is a high percentage of complete response to treatment, resulting in a high cure rate. Examples include Hodgkin's disease, and childhood and testicular cancers. Only 5 per cent of cancers fall into this group. The second group contains cancers that have a high complete response rate to chemotherapy, but a low cure rate. This group includes breast and ovarian cancers that may respond to drugs, prolonging life for months or years for some patients. The final group has a low response rate and low cure rate – chemotherapy is not very beneficial. Cancers in this group include prostate, pancreas, colon and stomach (McVie *et al* 2004). There is a small amount of palliation, and survival is typically increased by months rather than years.

There are currently more than 2,000 cancer drugs in development, and some drugs with specific molecular targets (biological or immunotherapies) are already available. They include trastuzumab (Herceptin, a monoclonal antibody that targets the HER-2 protein over-expressed in 20 to 25 per cent of breast cancers), imatinib (Gleevec, a growth inhibitor used in the treatment of chronic myeloid leukaemia and gastro-intestinal stromal tumours) and erlotinib (Tarceva, an epidermal growth factor inhibitor used as a second-line treatment and for recurrent non-small cell lung cancers).

Although these drugs have some clinical effect, their impact on survival may be marginal. This was demonstrated by the TRIBUTE trial, which compared the survival of patients with non-small cell lung cancer treated with erlotinib+carboplatin+paclitaxel with controls treated with placebo+carboplatin+paclitaxel. The median survival for patients treated with erlotinib was 10.6 months compared with 10.5 months for placebo (Herbst *et al* 2005).

However, the clinical effectiveness of new drugs may improve if developments in pharmacogenetics (the emerging science that studies how an individual reacts to a drug according to their genetic make-up) can be used to target the drugs to people who will benefit most.

It is possible that the new generation of cancer drugs that is now emerging will make the experience of cancer patients more like the experience of those with other chronic diseases. Biological therapies may keep the condition under control. A growing proportion of people will still be alive tens of years after their initial diagnosis, living in remission or with controlled metastatic disease. More and more people, in other words, will live long lives as cancer survivors.

The future of cancer surgery[8]

One of the major developments predicted for cancer surgery is computer-assisted surgery with three-dimensional imaging (Bhattacharya *et al* 2004). This may allow the tumour and anatomy of the organ to be clearly visible on a screen in front of the surgeon before the first cut is made, helping them to excise the tumour very precisely. Intra-operative diagnosis will also be more prevalent. Ultrasound scans used during surgery may show previously undiscovered metastases, which can be dealt with immediately.

Other possible imaging developments include marking tumours with a radioactive isotope, so that a Geiger counter passed over the body can detect distant metastases, or with fluorescent markers that glow in the dark (Bhattacharya *et al* 2004). These developments are expected to occur within the next 20 years.

Adjunctive therapies will be used at the same time as surgery. The area surrounding the tumour can be irradiated during the operation or chemotherapy drugs injected into blood vessels to prevent any cancer cells 'escaping' (chemoembolisation). Already, chemotherapy is used to shrink tumours before they are removed, followed by more chemotherapy or radiotherapy to prevent reoccurrence (Bhattacharya *et al* 2004). Use of preventive surgery could become more prevalent as screening tests become more advanced, and those at high risk will be identified earlier.

Patients will increasingly be cared for by organ-specific teams working in a small number of specialised centres. Team members will include surgeons, oncologists, pathologists and other allied health professionals. They will stay in hospital for less time, and many procedures will be carried out as day cases.

The high costs of increased technology will be offset by smaller amounts spent on long hospital stays and lower morbidity (illness). Post-operative patients will increasingly be cared for in the community and monitored by their team via email, telephone or video links (Bhattacharya et al 2004).

Other emerging technologies that may eventually transform treatment are on the more distant horizon. Robotic arms are already being used for operations. The surgeon operating the robot does not have to be physically in theatre, and could be in another city or even continent (Bhattacharya et al 2004).

Radiotherapy[9]

Radiotherapy can be used in combination with surgery and chemotherapy, and is especially effective in the treatment of prostate cancer. However, some experts predict that it will not be used in 20 years' time (Kunkler et al 2004) as it is undervalued and has suffered from long-term underinvestment. Although radiotherapy requires a high initial outlay, the cost per treatment is low.

Improvements in functional imaging will go hand in hand with developments in radiotherapy delivery. Positron emission tomography (PET) scanning will provide information about the functional anatomy of a tumour so that radiotherapy can be targeted very precisely. Intensity modulated radiotherapy shapes a beam of radiation very precisely so that healthy tissue is spared as much as possible. Combining this with PET scanning during treatment (rather than scanning after treatment is finished, as happens now) will save patients from unnecessary toxicity as treatment can be stopped early if it is not working (Bosanquet and Sikora 2006).

Other more speculative technological developments include the robotic 'cyperknife' which combines a linear accelerator with a computerised tomography (CT) scanner, delivering radiotherapy from six different angles.

Boron neutron capture is a technique that can be used to deliver radiation from within a tumour. Boron can be added to drugs that are taken up by tumours and then irradiated with a low energy neutron beam; this is biologically targeted radiation (Bosanquet and Sikora 2006). These futuristic sounding developments are currently being used in other countries.

There are staffing implications for these technological innovations. The skill mix of the cancer care team may need to be adjusted. Retention also needs to be improved, and more radiographers will need to be trained.

Summary

There is little doubt that the technology of cancer care will continue to develop, reflecting the large sums of money spent worldwide on research and development.

What is less clear is the timescale over which these developments will have a significant impact on survival, how they will impact on the overall burden of cancer and what they will mean for the way that cancer services are provided.

The next section outlines some of the views of our interviewees on these issues, and their thoughts on the future organisation of cancer services.

5 Summary of interview findings

We conducted ten interviews with experts in different aspects of cancer epidemiology, treatment and organisation (*see* the Appendix) to explore their views on:

- the impact of the Cancer Plan
- the organisation of cancer services
- patient priorities for the future
- key influences on the future need for and supply of cancer services, including epidemiological trends and the potential impact of new technologies
- the prevention and early detection of cancer and the balance between preventive and treatment services
- the process for reviewing and developing cancer policy
- the potential content of future cancer policy.

The interviewees are not necessarily representative of all available views on cancer.

A core interview schedule was developed covering these themes, and supplemented with additional questions to reflect the specific knowledge and expertise of each interviewee and to test our emerging ideas about future cancer policy.

Some interviewees wanted their remarks to remain unattributed, so this section presents a summary of comments, plus unattributed quotes to explain and amplify the points made.

Views on the Cancer Plan

There was near-universal agreement among our interviewees that the Cancer Plan has been a 'good thing'; that it has raised the profile of cancer among policy-makers and made it more of a priority in the NHS.

There was also general agreement that it has provided a clear strategic direction for service developments, led to more streamlined clinical pathways, contributed to better access and shorter waiting times, improved treatment and survival rates, and encouraged a better experience for patients.

The Cancer Plan has created a road map – without which no progress would have been made.

Overall the Cancer Plan has been a good thing. It has improved access to services, speeded up patient journeys... and improved communication with patients.

There was universal support for the 'hub and spoke' model of service organisation brought in by the Cancer Plan, with specialist centres supporting peripheral generalist providers (*see* Section 7). Indeed, one interviewee described this networked approach as 'essential' where care is provided by many different providers.

However, many had serious concerns about the strategic and planning roles of cancer networks and the extent to which they can function effectively in a changing policy environment which are discussed further below.

There was also less agreement about the development of multidisciplinary teams. A few interviewees strongly supported these for bringing together disparate clinicians to co-ordinate clinical management planning. Others saw them as important in some cases but often unnecessary for patients with 'routine', uncomplicated cancers and therefore inefficient.

Some interviewees also expressed a general reservation that while the aspirations of the Cancer Plan were very good, there have been difficulties in implementing it. Many possible explanations for this were offered including arrangements for the allocation of resources and responsibility for implementation.

> *It's hard to roll out national projects because a lot of the money and responsibility has been devolved locally.*

Other concerns included the lack of guidance on measuring the impact of cancer services. The need for rapid methodological progress with outcomes measurement and adjusting for case mix and co-morbidity was also noted.

> *[The] idea of providing cancer outcome data was inherent in the Cancer Plan but this has not happened – apart from out-of-date cancer survival data from the cancer registries.*

> *It's hard to get risk-adjusted outcomes. It's taken the cardiac surgeons five years to put this kind of information in the public domain; there are only a few of them, and they had the incentive of Bristol to drive them… We need to record disease stage at presentation and co-morbidity to allow for case mix adjustment.*

Prevention and early detection

Some interviewees thought the Cancer Plan paid too little attention to preventing cancer.

> *Prevention has not been so effective. Screening and smoking cessation was left to PCTs [primary care trusts] rather than to the networks, so it hasn't been effective as it could have been.*

Two interviewees also noted continuing inequalities in the distribution of cancer risk (discussed in Section 2) and felt more should be done to tackle them.

> *You need multidimensional health intervention polices in areas of high social deprivation. There are all sorts of economic issues. Can you disentangle health interventions from genuine economic hardships? Without tackling economic problems can you affect health?*

However, others felt the balance struck between prevention and treatment may have been appropriate, given the limited range of cancer prevention interventions of proven effectiveness.

> *The only important prevention area is smoking cessation. The government is too slow in developing anti-smoking policy. All other prevention work is insignificant in comparison.*

> *There is lots of research under way on diet and cancer. But can we bring bowel cancer under control by primary prevention? Who knows?*

Several interviewees argued that we need to know more about what works in terms of behavioural change – and there is an active programme of government-funded research in this area. However, one interviewee argued that within five to ten years, developments in genetic risk banding (the identification of low penetrance genes that shape personal risk) will enable us to personalise prevention and develop highly individualised behaviour programmes and risk reduction plans (the 'technology' of prevention is also discussed in Section 4).

High-cost drugs

There was universal agreement that the slow trickle of new cancer drugs seen in recent years (and discussed in Section 4) will speed up, and that each launch will require hard decisions to be made about funding and eligibility for treatment. There was also general concern that the media's tendency to portray new drugs as 'miracle cures' is fuelling patient expectations and risks undermining the doctor–patient relationship.

> *The media are often unhelpful – they pronounce products as miracle drugs when in fact they lead to just a small increase in life expectancy. This creates false expectations.*

> *Patients are going to have to accept rationing. There will be hard choices to be made and patients and the public need to be involved, but from a position of understanding. This will require the provision of information in understandable ways, including [information] addressing non-English speaking and illiterate populations.*

However, two interviewees noted that the cost of new drugs is relatively small in comparison with the efficiency savings that could be made by redesigning pathways of care. For example, one noted that many of the estimated 17,000 NHS inpatients each day receiving cancer therapies could be treated in alternative settings. Another argued that as new chemotherapeutic agents emerge, less surgery will be needed and it will be possible to provide more treatment in day case or community facilities, with the savings re-directed towards the new drugs.

However, there was little consensus about the likely timescale for these developments. And some felt such changes would only delay public debate about how society wants to value each month of additional survival.

A few argued that explicit eligibility criteria will be needed, underpinned by information on effectiveness and public debate. In this context, there was both support for and concern about the work of the National Institute for Health and Clinical Excellence.

NICE is a great idea that works very badly... It takes two years longer than in other countries to get a decision and then it's not implemented quickly. The systematic review process wastes time; you just need to look at few key papers. It is unlikely that important findings, even if negative, would remain hidden.

If we want an equitable approach, based on NICE, for everyone, then there must be some delay.

Patient priorities for cancer care

Our interviewees recognised that emphasis on the two-week referral standard has speeded up access for patients referred via the cancer referral pathway. However, some argued that it has also distorted waiting times in other parts of the service.

The two-week wait target is a problem because it distorts waiting times for the investigation of other symptoms.

Despite, this, interviewees felt the patient pathway through cancer care does not need to be radically altered, although all felt it can still be speeded up and made more efficient.

Interviewees noted that gaps between health and social care, primary and secondary care and palliative care exist and need to be closed, although there were differences of opinion about how to do this. Suggestions included better clinical pathways and more effective multidisciplinary teams.

Interviewees also suggested that, from a patient's perspective, a range of developments are needed:

- better information at time of diagnosis and afterwards, including risk-adjusted outcome data on which to make choices
- more opportunities for informed, shared decision-making
- improved services in the community
- more and better day-care treatment
- improved palliative care services
- a dedicated key worker or lead clinician
- 24-hour a day access to specialist nurses and members of palliative care teams
- fair access to high-cost drugs.

Palliative care

Interviewees acknowledged some improvement in palliative care services and welcomed current activiy to implement the Gold Standards Framework for palliative care (Thomas 2003). Overall, they were seen as a relatively neglected area of cancer policy. A number mentioned the lack of resources directed at palliative care services.

Palliative and end-of-life services still have a long way to go. More resources are needed and there is still a low percentage of people dying at home. This will have to change with an ageing population.

One described the difficulties of moving different services together to create a critical mass for palliative care. Another pointed out the weak links between primary care, social care and palliative care providers. Three interviewees argued for the need to link the development of palliative care services to a wider debate about end-of-life care.

The changing context of cancer care

There was broad agreement that too much cancer care is provided in acute hospital inpatient facilities. Interviewees felt that ongoing surveillance of patients in remission does not require hospital facilities.

However, views differed about whether cancer should be seen in the same way as long-term conditions such as diabetes, heart disease and asthma. Some argued the outcome for many cancers is either death or cure. Very few (such a chronic myeloid leukaemia) are chronic. Most cancers follow a different pattern from long-term conditions.

We can learn from the chronic disease model but you can't apply it to cancer. I don't agree with description of cancer as chronic disease. Cancer has a chronicity. Patients may... live with [cancer] for 25 years or more, but have long periods when they are well. Many may eventually recur and once patients start dying they do so quite quickly. There is a different trajectory from other chronic diseases.

Others thought that cancers are like other chronic conditions – or may be for part of their clinical course. At these times, the aim is control rather than cure, although it was unclear whether this work should be done in primary or secondary care.

Of course cancer is a chronic disease. But this raises questions about whether it should be in primary care or secondary care... The [American] Kaiser [Permanente] model is the right way. We need a network of providers bringing in diverse services such as social care and transport.

Interviewees also argued that developments in diagnostics increasingly allow investigation in the community. Some also felt that the treatment of recurrence does not necessarily require further surgery and that palliative treatment can increasingly be provided in community settings. Several interviewees suggested that limited changes could be made now, building on lessons learned from other countries.

You need to look at the follow-up period between initial diagnosis and first relapse: it's currently in secondary care, but it should be in primary care. There should be a community-based service after patients have finished their first set of treatments, including a surveillance programme.

The UK has twice as many beds as other countries, we don't need so many. There should be an ambulatory model. Plurality of provision is important. We need to unbundle diagnostics and need to implement ambulatory, polyclinic models.

However, one other interviewee highlighted potential problems with losing the economies of scale associated with hospital care and another raised concerns about the financial arrangements for local drug delivery.

Things are stretched and difficult enough in hospital, with overflowing clinics. Out in the community would be much less efficient.

Chemo will be administered at home if it's affordable. In a quirk of the Treasury, chemo can be ordered VAT-free for delivery at home; although very few people do it. The price differential could be used to pay for home nursing.

Some interviewees were also concerned about whether there are enough skilled clinicians to implement such developments, and the likelihood of achieving sufficient 'buy in' from both primary and secondary care clinicians.

> *Transfer into the community will be hindered by the design of homes, lack of facilities, lack of informal carers, lack of support from community services such as physiotherapists and GPs. Nurses tend to see themselves as either hospital or community-based – they aren't good at bridging the two. We need more integration and understanding of the two roles.*

Research is needed to address these issues (*see* Section 7).

Choice and contestability

There was broad agreement that cancer services must respond to the patient 'choice' agenda (outlined in Section 6), and attempts by independent sector providers to enter the NHS cancer care market.

The need for 'empathic, honest information' to support choice was also noted, along with opportunities to talk with a health professional about available choices.

One interviewee saw new providers as a way of extending community care, but with provisos about the need for back-up from NHS hospitals. There was broad agreement that a 'mixed economy' of service providers is highly likely.

> *Some private companies are delivering chemotherapy at home. At first there were problems but it now works well, as they are effectively in shared care with NHS. We need to recognise that the NHS can no longer be the only provider.*

However, there were also concerns. Although most interviewees felt that cancer patients should not be denied choice, they also felt that most simply want the best treatment.

> *A small amount of competition between providers can improve services, but patients simply want the best treatment, not to have to choose between different providers. How can a patient choose between teams? This isn't a problem only for cancer patients, but is particularly acute for them.*

Some interviewees worried that excessive expansion of a market in cancer services provision could result in surplus capacity and reduced efficiency. They also felt the introduction of new providers could fragment and/or duplicate services, and that it could be hard to maintain expertise across multiple, smaller units.

One interviewee expressed a strong belief that if new providers are to enter the NHS market, they will have to participate in cancer networks and develop their services in line with local strategic objectives. Another described the potential for new networks that use IT and communications technologies to link disparate specialist centres with local providers.

> *We may in future see networks of providers that overlap geographically and compete. One would need to pull commissioners out of the networks... improve their skills and have them working alongside. This would allow different networks of providers to test*

out different ways of doing things... But having several competing providers could result in excess capacity and inefficiency.

Cancer networks

Commissioning issues

The effectiveness of cancer networks as they exist at present is partly determined by the role played by participating commissioners – and the commissioning ability of PCTs is variable.

Our interviewees felt that while some PCTs are leading the strategic direction of cancer networks, others lack the expert knowledge and skills needed to commission effectively, or find themselves in conflict with the priorities of cancer networks and large hospitals.

> *In [X County] the cancer network was a commissioning network. But in [Y City] the network has not been able to achieve commissioning. There is no buy in from commissioners. It is a talking shop only, it doesn't commission or provide so it's ineffective.*

Several interviewees argued that cancer commissioning should take place at supra-PCT level – either through clusters of PCTs or at national level. A care pathway approach was proposed as another way to strengthen commissioning, with commissioning strategies based on projected numbers for each cancer.

> *There are four levels of commissioning: practice-based commissioning; PCTs; supra-PCT; and specialist. Cancer should be commissioned at supra-PCT level, with rare cancers only commissioned at specialist level. At supra-PCT level there could be consortia... but these arrangements are not clear yet.*

Organisational issues

It will already be clear that our interviewees had diverse views about cancer networks. Advocates were convinced that they are the best way to bring together and co-ordinate the work of multiple service providers. The most sceptical interviewee described networks as 'not fit for purpose' and 'costly strategic bodies that don't deliver'.

Views differed on the future organisation of networks. One interviewee thought they should stay largely as they are, but that the rules by which they operate must be tightened.

> *All parts of the country should be covered [by networks] and all provider organisations should have to join (including foundation trusts). There needs to be more prescriptive central guidance.*

Others argued that the integration of provision and commissioning in a single network is unsustainable and that commissioning should be separated. One proposed they should commission services from networks of providers like the US health maintenance organisation Kaiser Permanente, which buys services from a plurality of providers working to common pathways and standards.

> *The only way forward for the NHS is a commissioning network approach like Kaiser... with a consistent care pathway or orchestrated care providers and an agreed clinical model commissioned from a plurality of providers.*

Interviewees saw networks as potentially covering NHS, independent and voluntary sector providers as well and possibly also social care and other services.

Summary

The interviews revealed areas of consensus about the positive impact of the cancer plan and about its gaps and weaknesses. They also highlighted various differences of opinion. These include the value of preventive work; the implications of choice and new providers of cancer services; and the future form and function of networks. These themes will be considered in more detail in Section 7. Before that, Section 6 reviews wider changes in NHS policy that affect the development of cancer services.

6 Recent policy developments

The Cancer Plan was published soon after the launch of the NHS Plan in 2000 (Department of Health 2000b). Many of its aims mirrored those proposed for the NHS as a whole.

However, the blueprint for the wider NHS has changed substantially since then. Patient choice, foundation trusts, competition between providers and new financial arrangements have significantly changed the landscape in which cancer services are provided.

In this section, we review recent policy developments and briefly explore their impact on cancer services. In the following section we consider their implication for the future development of cancer policy.

Changes in the high-level policy context

When the Cancer Plan was published, the government had just launched the largest and most fundamental reform programme that the NHS had ever experienced. That programme, set out in *The NHS Plan* (Department of Health 2000b), embodied many wide-ranging goals and specific targets – including targets for waiting times – set by the Department of Health. It was enforced by a rigorous system of performance management.

Although the origins of the Cancer Plan predate the NHS Plan, its underlying philosophy was compatible with it: a serious shortfall in performance had been identified and a nationally directed programme of improvement, expressed in terms of targets and working through a single broad approach to service configuration, was put in place to remedy it.

Some two years later, however, the government began to retreat from the 'top-down' approach to reforming the NHS in the face of strong criticisms from within and without the service. The critics argued that the use of targets was excessive and that the vast range of policies being introduced was sometimes inconsistent. For these reasons, they argued that the role of the Department of Health should be reduced.

From 2002 onwards, the government began to introduce a range of policies designed to free the local NHS from central government control and, at the same time, give users more influence over its operation. The Department of Health also accepted that the number of centrally determined targets should be reduced. This new direction of policy has come to comprise several elements.

CHOICE

The government introduced its patient choice programme to help reduce waiting lists by allowing patients to choose hospitals where waits were shorter. It has subsequently sought to create choice more widely, as part of its general policy of giving users a greater say in how services are delivered.

FOUNDATION TRUSTS

Foundation status frees trusts from the direct control of the Secretary of State. They have greater borrowing powers than other types of trust, giving them more scope to develop their services without reference to other parts of the NHS.

FINANCIAL REFORM

To support the introduction of patient choice for elective care, the government is reforming the way that hospital services are financed. The new system is called Payment by Results and it is based on a national tariff that sets fixed prices for all hospital treatments and procedures on an episode-by-episode basis.

It provides more levers to change the balance of services than block contracts, as the type and location of services can be encouraged or discouraged by setting a high or low tariff.

COMMISSIONING REFORM

The government is introducing two reforms of commissioning. The first is a reduction in the number of primary care trusts (PCTs) to create commissioners with more buying power in relation to provider trusts. The second is practice-based commissioning, which is intended to make purchasing more effective at local level by engaging clinicians in commissioning decisions.

NEW PROVIDERS

Initially, the government began to introduce new providers of elective care to the NHS in order to increase its capacity and has continued with this policy to create a degree of competition. It has gone on to indicate its support for introducing new providers across all NHS services, including those outside hospitals.

Overall, in the new version of the NHS being created, the drivers for change are to be a combination of 'market' type pressures and a regulatory structure designed to identify and respond to poor performance.

Tensions and complementarities

In some areas the policy developments set out above have worked with the grain of the Cancer Plan. This is particularly true of those in the Public Health White Paper *Choosing Health: Making healthier choices easier* (Department of Health 2004b), where initiatives to support the preventive measures set out in the Cancer Plan were reinforced.

In other areas, there are potential tensions between the philosophy of the Cancer Plan and that implicit in the new NHS, and these will become stronger as the new framework is developed.

■ Although the Cancer Plan has not been managed centrally on a day-to-day basis, it is overseen nationally and it embodies a single broad strategy of service development.

The philosophy of the new NHS is supportive of local initiative, rather than national planning. Implicit in this would be greater local discretion for PCTs to set their own cancer policy.

- The main focus of the Cancer Plan was to improve the organisation of hospital-based care. The new emphasis is on shifting care to the community.

- The new financial regime of Payment by Results was designed initially for elective/episodic care from a single provider, rather than the long patient journeys typical of cancer, and for hospital services rather than community ones. The cancer services provided by multiple networked providers do not fit easily with this payment system.

- The creation of foundation trusts was explicitly designed to encourage independent action, rather than the co-operation implicit in the concept of a cancer network.

- Encouragement of new providers, for profit and not-for-profit, also threatens the co-operative working implicit in the patient pathway and cancer networks. The pursuit of independent organisational goals may conflict with the collective objectives of the networks.

Impacts

These broad changes in the policy environment are already affecting the organisation and delivery of cancer services.

This can be seen from a recent review of the incentives acting on a single strategic health authority, which was conducted to explore the tensions and complementarities created by policy since the NHS Plan (Grant 2005).

The review included a case study of cancer services and identified concerns about many of the issues we have discussed here, including the impact of choice and the need to clearly identify where policy needs to be made nationally and where there is scope for local action. Its findings are summarised in the box overleaf.

Other examples of changes driven by recent reform include an NHS contract with US-based independent provider Ovations Healthcare to develop the primary care cancer workforce (Department of Health 2004d) and the UK independent provider Healthcare at Home providing home chemotherapy to NHS patients.

The drive for more community-based care

Two of the main 'market-type' drivers for change, mentioned above, are the financial incentives associated with Payment by Results and practice-based commissioning. The former encourages hospitals and other specialist providers to maximise any activity they can provide at a cost that is below the national tariff. The latter will provide incentives for GPs to reduce hospital referrals and manage patients in community settings (at presumed lower cost than hospital care).

At present the national tariff covers episodes of care that could be split between hospital and community settings. Work to 'unbundle' payment for care in different settings has not yet been implemented, so incentives remain to retain care in hospital settings.

SUMMARY OF CASE STUDY OF THE IMPACT OF CURRENT POLICY AND INCENTIVES ON THE SOUTH EAST LONDON CANCER NETWORK

Drawing on a combination of interviews and document analysis, this case study found that those involved in the cancer network considered collaborative working essential to success.

Policy that promotes competition and independent action was seen to jeopardise collaboration and to reinforce the boundaries between organisations. It was also seen to increase the risk of takeover by strong providers, at the possible cost of the loss of locally responsive services.

The current incentives environment was not effectively promoting an appropriate balance between primary, community and hospital services.

The case study commented that collaboration between specialist and other providers needs to pursue various objectives in tandem. These include localness, responsiveness and quality. It also noted that a strong commissioner would be needed to achieve this.

The study suggested that clinician-led multidisciplinary teams should be the focal point of collaboration and that local accessibility could be maintained through developing more community cancer services.

It also suggested that greater autonomy for cancer networks is essential to allow them to implement national initiatives and 'translate' them to fit the local context.

It concluded that a more sophisticated payment system is required with tariffs that reflect the complexity of cancer care. These should incentivise the implementation of agreed clinical pathways and the provision of selected services in local settings.

The report also concluded there is a need to distinguish two elements of commissioning that can be separated. First, the planning and design of services that can be done at national level (it argued that 80 to 90 per cent of patient pathways can be standardised, as can quality standards). Second, local contracting to specify how, where and by whom services should be provided locally.

The case study also concluded that the role of networks as either purchaser or providers of care should be clarified. Financial arrangements must be developed to support the chosen role.

(Source: Grant 2005)

Given the recognised weaknesses in commissioning, relatively powerful hospitals are able to resist commissioners' efforts to transfer services to community settings. In due course, hospitals may seek to take over provision of community services if they can provide them more cheaply than equivalent hospital services and below tariff rates. The tensions between the incentives built into Payment by Results and the wider government vision of providing more health care outside hospital are, in other words, substantial.

In response, the government published a White Paper, *Our Health, Our Care, Our Say* (Department of Health 2006c), that sets out its vision for the future configuration of English health services.

The four main goals of the White Paper are:

- health promotion, more effective prevention and earlier intervention

- transfer of services from acute hospitals to community settings

- reduced inequalities and improved access to general practice and other community health services

- better support for people with long-term conditions, including the major development of self-care programmes.

The White Paper makes little specific reference to cancer services, but the overall direction of travel that it sets out is highly relevant. Some of the main developments it proposes are:

- more specialist care provided in community settings, with initiatives to define clinically safe patient pathways to support this

- investment in new community facilities (sometimes termed 'polyclinics'), combining general practice, primary care, diagnostics and minor treatment

- a duty of partnership between health and social care to improve service integration for people with complex, chronic health problems

- patient empowerment for self-care including better access to information and care plans

- workforce development to support people with ongoing needs.

Tensions and complementarities

These proposals are largely consistent with the needs of cancer patients. For example, developing better access to information is already in progress in relation to cancer.

The development of clinical pathways around which to provide services is a central theme of the Cancer Plan. The vision described by some interviewees of more diagnosis and treatment in the community (*see* Section 5) will be supported by the White Paper.

Our Health, Our Care, Our Say also promises to encourage innovation and to support the introduction of new providers of primary care services. Again, these proposals are consistent with ideas put forward by our interviewees about new providers of cancer services.

Summary

The policy environment has changed substantially since the Cancer Plan was published. Patient choice and Payment by Results, the introduction of foundation trusts and new, private sector providers, all point towards a more 'market'-orientated NHS than was envisaged by its authors.

At the same time, the recent White Paper *Our Health, Our Care, Our Say,* presages a shift from hospital to community services.

Some of these changes work in tandem with existing cancer policy, and may push developments that are already under way. Others have the potential to be in tension with the current direction of cancer services. These issues are explored in more detail in the concluding section.

7 The next steps

Why the NHS Cancer Plan needs to be revised

The NHS Cancer Plan was one of the first of its kind, and its approach has been adopted for a number of other conditions and diseases, for instance, national service frameworks in coronary heart disease, mental health, diabetes and long-term conditions.

It has achieved considerable success in many areas. As Sections 1 and 2 show, cancer prevention has been addressed through smoking-cessation services and programmes to encourage children and adults to eat more fruit and vegetables. Screening programmes have also been extended.

Cancer networks have been established. The speed of access to diagnosis and treatment has improved for patients who are referred through the two-week referral pathway. Additional cancer specialists have been recruited and specialist multidisciplinary teams set up. There has been considerable investment in diagnostic and treatment facilities, and some steps have been taken to improve palliative care services.

However, Sections 1 and 2 also show there are gaps in the Cancer Plan and that further progress needs to be made. The National Audit Office has raised concerns about the lack of forecasting in the Cancer Plan, the lack of mechanisms for updating it and about the functioning of cancer networks.

The impact of the government's approach to prevention is unknown, and our interviewees were divided on the effort that should be put into this area of activity. Many patients are still not being referred as urgent cases, and some of our interviewees were concerned about the wider effects of the Cancer Plan's two-week waiting time target for urgent referrals.

There are ongoing concerns about access to diagnostic and radiotherapy services. The Royal College of Radiologists has shown that waiting times for radiotherapy have not improved as a result of the Cancer Plan. And our interviewees felt more attention could still be given to palliative care services and their integration with other community services.

In addition, Section 3 shows that demographic trends will increase the incidence of cancer in coming decades and that better treatments will increase the number of survivors. The inevitable effect is that more people will live with cancer in remission and this is bound to increase the demand for resources for cancer.

It also poses a challenge to services, which our interviewees felt are already too heavily focused on hospitals. In the future, there will be more scope to monitor and manage patients in the community; but considerable work is needed to determine the best models for doing this.

Section 4, meanwhile, demonstrates that prevention and treatment will not stand still. Prevention may become more effective and personalised; but the impact on cancer incidence and prevalence is unknown. Thousands of new cancer drugs are in development, but many are high cost and currently of marginal benefit. Our interviewees were concerned about media coverage of these new drugs, and argued that a national debate is needed on what should be provided to whom.

In Section 5, our interviewees also reflected on the effectiveness of cancer networks and on the likely impact of new policy developments, outlined in more detail in Section 6.

The policy environment has changed greatly since the Cancer Plan was published, with the arrival of foundation trusts, new private sector providers, patient choice and the new funding policy of Payment by Results. Our interviewees were unsure about the impact of these changes on networks, and work is needed to develop a 'network policy' for the future.

The environment in which cancer services operate and cancer policy is made, therefore, has changed since 2000 and will continue to do so. This is already leading to tensions around prevention, access to treatment, and the role of new providers.

The merits of a smoking ban in public places, 'traffic light' food labelling and restricting the advertising of 'junk food' are all highly contested. The very public demands made by some breast cancer patients for Herceptin may well be repeated for other drugs in the coming years.

Private sector providers of chemotherapy and long-term care have entered the health care market, but their role and links to NHS provision is, as yet, unclear.

For all these reasons, we need to revisit the Cancer Plan and cancer policy, to build on progress, fill gaps, and start to prepare for the changes that the trends in epidemiology, technology and policy explored in this report will bring about.

In the rest of this section, we identify and discuss three broad areas where further policy will be most helpful:

- addressing gaps and weaknesses in the coverage and scope of the Cancer Plan
- revising the role of networks
- examining the scope, costs and benefits of shifting care to community settings.

Gaps and weaknesses

As noted above, a series of gaps and weaknesses in the current Cancer Plan have been identified throughout this report. These include areas where policy was either absent or needs to be strengthened and areas of incomplete implementation.

Baseline knowledge and information

The first gap (identified in the National Audit Office (NAO) report (2005b) discussed in Section 1 and by interviewees in Section 5) is the knowledge and information on which cancer policy is based and through which it is monitored.

This preliminary work is particularly important since the trends in incidence, survival and prevalence discussed in Section 3 will increase the number of people needing care. At the same time the resources available for service improvement are likely to be in short supply, if, as is widely anticipated, the rapid rate of growth in the NHS budget triggered in 2000 begins to level off in two years' time.

Guidance from the World Health Organization (WHO 2002) says that the first stage of any policy revision should be detailed modelling of future demands for care and of the resources needed to provide it.

There is also a need to model the potential impact of changes in risk factors, in preventive policies (demands) and in current capacity (supply). This work should be undertaken now as a starting point for future policy development.

Equally important will be the development and implementation of outcome measures for cancer services that allow the impact of policy changes, higher spending levels and new forms of treatment to be identified.

The methodological challenges associated with outcomes measurement were not explored in detail in this report. However, the importance of developing better information on performance and outcomes to inform patient choice was noted. This information is also required to monitor the impact of service developments driven by other areas of health policy, including those outlined in Section 6.

Therefore, an interim set of outcome measures should be developed, backed up by a research programme to refine adjustment for case mix and co-morbidity.

Balancing prevention and treatment

A second perceived weakness in the Cancer Plan, raised particularly by our interviewees (*see* Section 5), is an imbalance between its focus on developing acute sector services and cancer treatment and its relatively limited focus on prevention, early detection and palliation.

Aside from further reducing tobacco consumption, our interviewees had mixed views on the value of developing preventive services, although one of the NAO reports (NAO 2005b), claimed there was strong support for more emphasis on prevention.

The NAO report also noted the need for better understanding of the factors leading to continued delays in access to care. We identified this issue in Section 3 as partly explaining the relatively poor performance of NHS cancer services.

Significant socio-demographic variations still exist in the distribution of risk factors, in awareness of cancer symptoms and in help-seeking behaviour (as well as in cancer incidence and mortality).

Reducing such inequalities was a primary aim of the Cancer Plan. But it is not clear where the balance should lie between campaigns to increase knowledge and awareness of cancer symptoms and efforts to improve the cultural sensitivity and appropriateness of services.

Some 'spearhead' primary care trusts (PCTs) (the most deprived PCTs in the country) are exploring how to raise awareness about cancer (House of Commons 2005). But such projects are typically small scale and not part of a wider strategy for prevention and early detection. Similarly, it is not clear how efforts to reduce inequalities in risk factors for and the incidence of cancer link into other NHS initiatives to reduce health inequalities more broadly.

More research into these issues is still needed if future cancer policy is to address continued inequalities and improve early presentation and diagnosis effectively.

Balancing treatment and palliation

Palliative care services are improving, but their development has been relatively neglected during implementation of the Cancer Plan. One of the NAO reports discussed earlier found that, in some cases, patient experience remained poor (NAO 2005a).

Some of our interviewees felt that resources for palliative care had been limited and that limited progress had been made with integrating palliative services with primary and community care. This is beginning to change with the implementation of the Gold Standards Framework for palliative care (Thomas 2005). But much more is still needed.

Several other areas of current health policy also support the further development of palliative care services. These include the broad vision set out in the White Paper *Our Health, Our Care, Our Say* (Department of Health 2006c) to transfer care into the community (*see* Section 6) and the scope for patient choice to support choice of place of death. The growth of independent and voluntary sector providers may also increase the diversity of end-of-life services in community settings.

In addition, initiatives now under way to improve services for people with long-term conditions may also contribute to a new focus on palliative care. Many cancer patients are living with other conditions such as heart failure and lung disease, so controlling their cancer symptoms forms part of their complex health and social care needs. The emerging role of community matrons as case managers and co-ordinators between different service providers may well have spin-off effects on palliative care.

Any revision of cancer policy must harness these changes in the wider policy environment to encourage real innovation in palliative care services. Their development should also be linked to wider developments in the management of complex, chronic illness.

This will mean additional requirements for workforce development and support for better integration between different community providers; issues discussed further below, in relation to shifting care to community settings.

Guidance on high-cost drugs

A third perceived gap in the Cancer Plan relates to policy and guidance on new and emerging therapies, and in particular high-cost drugs.

In Section 3, we described the epidemiological trends that underlie the rising prevalence of people living with a cancer diagnosis. In Section 4, we outlined areas in which improved treatments are most likely to contribute to improved survival.

These trends will increase the proportion of patients who experience a relapse who could benefit from high-cost cancer drugs. As we have already pointed out, a significant growth in demand for these treatments – however marginal the benefits – is inevitable, although advances in genetic technology and 'personalised' prescribing may enable us to target these drugs at the people who will benefit most.

Interviewees anticipated a significant increase in the rate at which expensive new cancer drugs are launched. They were also united in anticipating rising patient expectations of access to these drugs – fuelled by media coverage – and seeing a need for future policy to address issues of access and eligibility.

In one sense, these issues were dealt with when the Secretary of State for Health announced that Herceptin would be available to all NHS patients, if clinically appropriate (Department of Health 2005b). The announcement by-passed the usual NICE approval process. However, the opportunity costs of this announcement within cash-strapped PCTs will be significant. And it raises questions – illustrated in the differing opinions of our interviewees – about the ongoing suitability of the NICE approval process.

A revision of cancer policy must tackle these difficult issues. A number of preliminary steps are needed to support this process:

- we need to apply the activity modelling referred to above to alternative clinical pathways, so as to identify potential efficiency savings from different patterns of care. For example, the argument put forward in Section 5 that new drugs cost relatively little in relation to hospital spending, and they could be afforded for the time being through efficiency savings, needs to be properly assessed

- we need more research and public debate about how to value the marginal gains in survival associated with new cancer drugs and how to assess the related opportunity costs to other cancer services and to the wider NHS

- we need to develop new mechanisms to involve patients and the public in decisions about high-cost cancer drugs. But it is not clear what these should be. Should they be at national level, either through the relatively indirect mechanism of participation in the NICE evaluation process, or through stakeholder involvement in re-shaping national cancer policy? Or should they be at local level, with public involvement in local policy-making and developing local criteria for clinical eligibility? Any future revision of cancer policy should work on how to do this.

Networks and cancer centres

The introduction of cancer networks attracted praise and condemnation in almost equal measure from our interviewees (*see* Section 5) and were seen as both a strength and a weakness of the Cancer Plan.

The third NAO report discussed in Section 1 (2005b) similarly credited them with significant achievements, while identifying areas for further development.

A review of the role of networks is particularly needed in response to the changing policy environment described in Section 6 (where some of the tensions with existing cancer policy were also raised).

Three options emerged from the literature review and interviews that informed this report:

- networks to continue in their current form, with improved functioning through tighter guidance and monitoring
- commissioning networks that commission services from multiple providers (that may also be networked)
- provider networks that bring together and co-ordinate services from multiple providers in response to commissioner specifications.

MAINTAINING CURRENT NETWORKS

Existing networks were praised for bringing different stakeholders together, and some have made real achievements. Failures were attributed to many causes, including under-resourcing of management teams, lack of senior manager involvement, variable relationships with PCTs and lack of formal agreement about ways of working (NAO 2005b).

These issues *could* be addressed through tighter rules that guarantee resources, senior manager attendance and so on. However, we do not believe this will *necessarily* result in more effective networks.

Given the incentives inherent in Payment by Results, network participants may be reluctant to suspend the wider objectives of their organisation if they clash with network goals.

In a recent review of networks, Nick Goodwin also cautions against over-regulation (Goodwin 2004). His study found that centrally directed goals were hard to implement at local level. Goodwin also cautioned against 'network capture' by strong institutional members. This problem was reported by some interviewees, who felt that large hospitals or well-organised purchasers dominated their local networks. It was also highlighted by the NAO (NAO 2005b).

In Section 6 we described the incentives on foundation trusts to extend their services and noted that network capture could facilitate this. We also described the limited capacity of most commissioners to challenge providers. In these circumstances it is hard to be confident that tighter central guidance and regulation will result in more effective networks.

COMMISSIONING NETWORKS

Some interviewees argued that commissioning should be separated from provision and that commissioners should form networks themselves. In one sense, the NAO found this is already happening. Some clusters of PCTs are identifying a 'lead commissioner' and agreeing to fund a common cancer strategy – albeit through current cancer networks.

These arrangements are similar to those which emerged for other areas of specialist commissioning within the NHS internal market in the 1990s. Some 'commissioning consortia' worked well and were able to pool resources to assess need and plan service provision. But others ran into difficulties (Stern 1995). Problems arose if the common strategy of the consortium conflicted with other local goals and if funding commitments were required that exceeded a participant's ability to pay.

Two of our interviewees proposed the idea of specialist, supra-PCT commissioners. It would be possible to develop free-standing, cancer commissioning organisations with top-sliced funding – but this would reduce local influence over cancer services, going against the spirit of much current policy.

An additional problem with this approach lies in the absence of reliable outcome and performance measures. Commissioning networks would be in a weak position to monitor the performance and quality of services they obtain.

As PCTs start to merge, there may be new opportunities to review and strengthen cancer commissioning. Enhancing the skills and knowledge needed to commission cancer services is a key development priority; and one that will become even more pressing if PCT reorganisation instead displaces existing commissioning staff with expertise and local knowledge of cancer services.

Clear thinking is required about the levers available to steer the strategic development of cancer services and to strengthen them (these may include contracts, incentives, regulations and targets). Clear thinking is also needed about how to unbundle the national tariff brought in by Payment by Results, to create aligned incentives across primary and secondary care.

PROVIDER NETWORKS

Provider networks are already in place through the hub and spoke arrangements for cancer services. But current policy to develop market-type incentives creates an opportunity for new forms of network to emerge.

Again, there are many potential options. Networks could remain geographically bound, as they are now, bringing together generalist and site-specific specialist cancer services, palliative care and preventive work. In time, and if community-based cancer services expand, they may also incorporate other primary, community and social care providers.

Alternatively, policies to promote choice and competition could encourage the emergence of competing networks, in which digital and information technologies link geographically dispersed specialist centres with local providers.

In this case, the potential benefits are increased patient choice and competitive incentives to increase operational efficiency – but the potential risks include developing excess capacity in cancer services and whole-system inefficiency.

Network capture by large powerful providers is also a problem in provider-only networks. It would be up to commissioners to prevent this from happening, if it jeopardised the provision of services that respond to patient preferences and needs. Commissioners would also need to ensure that a shift to community-based services takes place (see below). As discussed, it is unclear, at present, what proportion of commissioners could manage this.

Overall, options must be identified for developing a 'network policy' and a coherent intellectual basis for how non-institutionalised collaboration can work in the face of choice and competition.

Commissioners could have a key role in this process. But it is not clear whether they would be able in practice to introduce, monitor and regulate new providers. Can commissioners develop the skills to act as effective market-makers? If not, what should this mean for the emerging mixed economy of service providers?

The scope, cost and benefits of shifting to community settings

The possibility of providing more cancer care in the community has been a recurrent theme throughout this report. Reasons for this include:

- epidemiological trends, which mean more people will be living with cancer in remission in the future

- emerging technologies allowing more to be done in the community

- the need to reduce the costs of hospital care to fund high-cost drugs and other cancer services

- the high use of hospital facilities in England compared with other countries

- wider NHS policy promoting the provision of more services in community settings.

A number of important questions must be addressed to guide the future development of community-based cancer services.

First, should cancer be considered in the same way as long-term conditions?

The summary of epidemiological trends in Section 3 highlighted the trends that will lead to more people living with cancer in remission. But our interviewees were divided about the implications for how cancer should be seen.

Some felt that many people are perfectly well in remission, and need to be vigilant for symptoms of recurrence, rather than regularly reviewed. Others felt people with advanced cancer have the same complex health and social care problems as those with other long-term conditions, so a similar approach may be appropriate.

This gives rise to a second question: How appropriate would it be to link the development of community-based cancer services to parallel developments for people with long-term conditions? There is a growing cadre of 'community matrons' providing intensive support for older people with multiple, complex chronic conditions, many of whom are also at high risk of cancer.

Can they make a useful contribution to cancer care alongside specialist palliative care teams? What will be the best way to co-ordinate the provision of community-based services for cancer with other services for long-term conditions to avoid duplication and fragmentation?

Third, Section 4 discussed some of the technological developments that may support community-based services, but our interviewees were unclear about the timeframe over which these developments will occur. One interviewee pointed out that emerging drug treatments remain complex to administer. The cost-effectiveness of providing different forms of chemotherapy in the community remains unclear.

Fourth, what developments are required in workforce and in facilities to support more cancer care in the community? The Cancer Plan stimulated workforce development initiatives for palliative care. But how well equipped are GPs and existing community clinicians to monitor cancer patients, detect signs of recurrence and co-manage symptoms and side effects in collaboration with specialists?

Will the development of polyclinics and community hospitals proposed in the White Paper *Our Health, Our Care, Our Say* (Department of Health 2006c) provide the necessary facilities for diagnosis and treatment in the community? Through what process should potential developments be reviewed, modelled and planned?

Fifth, how far should the development of local, community-based services be pursued in relation to cancer services? The rhetoric of the White Paper is about localness, responsiveness and convenience. But there is strong evidence in favour of concentrating expertise in centres of excellence. Explicit debate is needed about how to balance these aspirations and the implications for developing services in the community.

Developing policy on the shift to community services

Although government policy as a whole supports a shift in the balance of care across a broad spectrum of services, the costs and benefits of such a shift in cancer services have yet to be worked out in detail, as the questions raised above show. We propose a series of activities to support policy development:

- different future scenarios for community-based cancer services should be developed, with associated modelling of potential needs and costs. These should, where possible, inform the design of facilities and services developed in response to the White Paper, to ensure the opportunity for developing cancer services in the community is not missed

- pilot services should be developed to explore the advantages and disadvantages of linking palliative care with other wider developments in services for complex, chronic illness

- alternative models for community service should be developed, piloted and evaluated before being rolled out nationally

- work should be done to ensure the compatibility – or otherwise – of these models with the current financial framework and, if required, to develop new financial systems (such as unbundled tariffs) that support a change in the balance of care

- a workforce development strategy is required to support developments in community-based services

- public debate should be encouraged on the balance between local and convenient services and centres of excellence.

In short, if community-based cancer services are to develop in response to the factors discussed in this report, the appropriate payment system, targets, guidelines and other incentives must be in place.

The process for revising cancer policy

The time for a 'once and for all' cancer plan is past. As the earlier sections of this report have made clear, the cancer environment is rapidly changing and the coming years are likely to experience more – rather than less – change.

It follows that the development of cancer policy from now on should be seen as a rolling process of research and policy analysis. It should include experimentation with, and piloting of, new ideas, particularly in developing new models of care for community-based services.

How should the work be led and directed?

Localism is a key theme in current NHS policy (Reid 2003). Local decision-making, local accountability and greater local responsiveness are all set to increase. The logic of applying this approach to cancer services would be that PCTs, or groups of PCTs, would be left in charge of developing cancer policy in collaboration with the provider networks they commission from.

However, there will always be counter-pressures. Public concern about postcode prescribing, for example, is directed at national politicians, who are popularly regarded as being in charge of the health service. Even if localities are given greater scope to develop policies of their own and experiment with new models of care for community services, responsibility for the overall policy and financial framework will still lie with the centre. Equally, much of the research agenda is best seen as a national responsibility, since the main issues to be addressed arise in all parts of the country.

Therefore, we believe that a revision of the Cancer Plan and development of new cancer policy should be the responsibility of a cancer policy group within the Department of Health, led by the National Cancer Director.

Nevertheless, the revision process should involve all stakeholders (both professionals and users) and it should be supported by substantial analytical and research resources both inside and outside the Department of Health.

Methods for stakeholder involvement should be developed that give a genuine voice to service users and their carers and to the growing array of service providers.

In the medium to long term, there is also a need to ensure that cancer research contributes more fundamentally to the development of cancer policy. A programme of research is needed to focus on the gaps already identified and others that emerge from the work priorities set out below.

What should be done?

We have identified many areas of work that are needed to clarify what direction future policy should take. In summary, we propose five areas that are particularly important in this respect:

- developing baseline knowledge for cancer policy and the strategic development of cancer services

- prioritising research to support policy and health service development
- addressing gaps and weaknesses in the current Cancer Plan
- clarifying options for the organisation and functions of cancer networks
- experimentation and evaluation in community-based cancer services.

Developing baseline knowledge

Throughout this paper, we have identified areas where information, analysis and modelling are required. These include analysis of need and demand and activity forecasting based on challenging assumptions about redesigning care pathways to reduce inpatient care. There is also a need to collect and analyse data on hospital adherence to clinical guidelines.

However, the pace of change in treatment and survival associated with new technologies is uncertain. This makes it hard to predict the rate of change of care pathways. Analysis of *potential* need, demand and activity based on different future scenarios should also be undertaken.

The research agenda

There is a need to define a clear research agenda for NHS cancer services and to give it far greater prominence than it currently enjoys in the national cancer research programme.

It will need at minimum to cover:

- research to support weak areas of the Cancer Plan, such as modifying risk behaviour, pain control and palliative care. Work is under way in relation to chronic disease management, and it will be important to draw on this learning

- research to define measures of success, the data collection needed to put them into practice, and the data needed to inform patient choice

- research into the clinical and cost-effectiveness and the acceptability of providing selected cancer services in the community.

Addressing gaps and weaknesses in the current Cancer Plan

In preparing this report, we have identified three areas where further policy guidance is particularly important in closing gaps in the existing Cancer Plan: reducing inequalities, rebalancing activity between prevention/early detection, treatment and palliation, and providing guidance on access to high-cost drugs.

The first two of these priority areas should be mutually supportive, given continuing inequalities in the distribution of risk factors and delayed presentation of symptoms. Nevertheless, policy in this area will need to be underpinned by judgements about how far to prioritise prevention given the weak evidence base and how far to prioritise resources for palliative care.

Other judgements are required in relation to access to high-cost drugs. We need a public debate, with informed media coverage, about how to value the marginal gains in survival associated with new cancer drugs.

Notwithstanding earlier comments about the limits to localism in relation to cancer policy, we call for new approaches to public and patient involvement in decisions about introducing new drugs, the local implementation of cancer policy and service configuration, and the increasingly complex ethical issues involved.

Clarifying options for the organisation and functions of cancer networks

Options must be identified for developing cancer networks, with a coherent intellectual basis for how non-institutionalised collaboration can work in the face of choice and competition. A coherent policy framework must be developed that reflects a decision about whether to strengthen current arrangements or develop separate purchaser and provider networks.

The policy framework will need to reflect the extent to which market incentives will be developed in relation to cancer services and the likely extent to which multiple new providers (whether for profit or voluntary sector) will be delivering cancer services. These issues are still being resolved within the wider NHS policy community. However, emerging policy on cancer networks should be informed by these factors as wider policy is made.

Work is also needed to establish what the most effective purchasing structure is likely to be and what the balance should be between, on the one hand, national specifications on the structure of cancer services and, on the other, allowing more local discretion to encourage innovation linked to evaluation.

Experimentation and evaluation in community-based cancer services

There is also a need for better understanding of service delivery options for long-term monitoring of people in remission and on long-term maintenance therapy. Important questions need to be resolved about the role that primary care can effectively fulfil, the workforce it would need to fulfil it, the likely cost of such developments and the combination of policy levers likely to bring them about.

Innovative developments should be encouraged in community-based cancer services. Attention should also be paid to how to engage primary and community clinicians to ensure they work effectively with specialist providers, and to other workforce initiatives that might be needed.

Alternative service models should be developed, piloted and evaluated before being spread nationally. It will also be necessary to ensure their compatibility – or otherwise – with the current financial framework and, if required, to develop new financial systems (such as unbundled tariffs) that support any necessary change in the balance of care.

Conclusion

We have outlined epidemiological trends that will increase the need for cancer services and technological trends that will drastically alter treatment options. We have also described the challenges of continuing to implement the NHS Cancer Plan in the changing policy environment. A review of policy is now required to address these challenges and prepare cancer services for a changing future. We present the ideas in this report to stimulate debate and action.

Appendix:
List of interviewees

Dr Jamie Ferguson
Consultant in Public Health Medicine and Lead in Cancer
Lambeth PCT

Professor David Forman
Director of Information and Research
Northern and Yorkshire Cancer Registry and Information Service
(*telephone interview*)

Jenny Grant
Service Delivery Manager
Haematology Clinic
Guy's and St Thomas' Hospital

Professor Roger James
Professor of Oncology and Director of Kent Cancer Services
The Kent Cancer Centre

Professor Peter Johnson
Cancer Research UK Professor of Medical Oncology
Southampton General Hospital

Dame Gill Oliver
Consultant to Macmillan Cancer Support

Professor Amanda Ramirez
Division of Cancer Studies
King's College London

Professor Mike Richards
National Cancer Director

Professor Karol Sikora
Scientific Director
Medical Solutions Plc

Professor Paul Workman
Professor of Pharmacology and Therapeutics
The Institute of Cancer Research
(*brief telephone interview*)

Endnotes

1 This figure is taken from the website www.cancerscreening.nhs.uk/breastscreen/

2 For further information go to www.goldstandardsframework.nhs.uk/ and www.lcp-mariecurie.org.uk/

3 Data reported under this subheading are taken from the Cancer Research UK website. For more information, go to http://info.cancerresearchuk.org/cancerstats/incidence/trends/?a=5441

4 Data reported under this subheading are taken from the Cancer Research UK website. For more information, go to http://info.cancerresearchuk.org/cancerstats/mortality/timetrends/?a=5441

5 Data reported under this subheading are taken from the government's Office of National Statistics website. For more information, go to www.statistics.gov.uk/CCI/nugget.asp?ID=861&Pos=3&ColRank=1&Rank=374

6 For more information about the UK Collaborative Trial of Ovarian Cancer Screening, go to www.ukctocs.org.uk/

7 For more information on the Dutch–Belgian controlled lung cancer screening trials, go to www.controlled-trials.com/isrctn/trial/%7C/0/63545820.html

8 This section has been developed using ideas from Bhattacharya *et al* (2004).

9 This section has been developed using ideas from Kunkler *et al* (2004) and Chapter 6 in Bosanquet and Sikora (2006).

Bibliography

Action on Smoking and Health (ASH) (2005). *Basic Facts 3 : Tobacco economics*. London: ASH. Available online at : www.ash.org.uk/html/factsheets/html/basic03.html (accessed on 16 June 2006).

Advisory Council on Breast Cancer Screening (2006). *Screening for Breast Cancer in England: Past and future*. Sheffield: NHS Cancer Screening Programmes.

American Cancer Society (2006). 'Early detection trial for current and former smokers'. Available online at: www.cancer.org/docroot/PED/content/PED_10_2x_National_Lung_Screening_Trial.asp (accessed on 27 June 2006).

Ash D, Barrett A, Hinks A, Squire C (2004). 'Audit of national waiting times for radiotherapy'. *Clinical Oncology*, vol 16, pp 387–94.

Bhattacharya S, McPherson S, Mokbel K (2004). 'Cancer 2025: surgery'. *Expert Review of Anticancer Therapy*, vol 4, 3s1, SS33–36.

Bosanquet N, Sikora K (2006). *The Economics of Cancer Care*. Cambridge: Cambridge University Press.

Bray F, Moller B (2006). 'Predicting the future burden of cancer'. *Nature Reviews Cancer,* vol 6, pp 63–74.

Cancer Research UK (2006). 'Vaccine to prevent HPV infection, the cause of cervical cancer, in women aged 26 years and over (HPV 015)'. Available online at: www.cancerhelp.org.uk/trials/trials/trial.asp?trialno=7491 (accessed on 27 June 2006).

Cancer Research UK (undated). 'Healthy living'. Available online at: http://info.cancerresearchuk.org/healthyliving/ (accessed on 27 June 2006).

Cancer Research UK (undated). 'UK Cervical Cancer Mortality Stratistics'. Available online at: http://info.cancerresearchuk.org/cancerstats/types/cervix/mortality/ (accessed on 11 July 2006).

Dalgleish A, Richards M, Sikora K (2004). 'Cancer 2025: prevention'. *Expert Review of Anticancer Therapy*, vol 4, 3s1, S19–23.

Department of Health (2006a). 'England Summary. Cancer waiting times: monitoring the one month wait target from diagnosis to treatment for all cancers'. Available online at: www.performance.doh.gov.uk/cancerwaits/2005/q3/part6.html (accessed on 27 June 2006).

Department of Health (2006b). *Cancer Waiting Times: England*. Available online at: www.performance.doh.gov.uk/cancerwaits/2005/q4/part6.html (accessed on 16 June 2006).

Department of Health (2006c). *Our Health, Our Care, Our Say*. London: The Stationery Office.

Department of Health (2005a). *Departmental Report 2004*. Cmnd 6204. London: The Stationery Office. Available online at: www.dh.gov.uk/assetRoot/04/08/12/85/04081285.pdf (accessed on 16 June 2006).

Department of Health (2005b). 'Hewitt fast tracks cancer drug to save 1,000 lives' (press release, 5 October 2005, 2005/0339). Available online at: www.dh.gov.uk/PublicationsAndStatistics/ PressReleases/PressReleasesNotices/fs/en?CONTENT_ID=4120630&chk=eihnMJ (accessed on 27 June 2006).

Department of Health (2005c). Investment in Cancer Services 2001/02 – 2003/04. Gateway reference 5447. London: Department of Health.

Department of Health (2004a). *Chief Executive's Report to the NHS*. London: The Stationery Office.

Department of Health (2004b). *Choosing Health: Making healthier choices easier*. London: The Stationery Office.

Department of Health (2004c). *The NHS Cancer Plan and the New NHS: Providing a patient-centred service*. London: Department of Health.

Department of Health (2004d). '£6 million for cancer care project' (press release 2004/0325). Available online at: www.dh.gov.uk/PublicationsAndStatistics/PressReleases/PressReleases Notices/fs/en?CONTENT_ID=4088999&chk=O3Yjyz (accessed on 27 June 2006).

Department of Health (2003). *NHS Cancer Plan. Three-year Progress Report: Maintaining the momentum*. London: Department of Health.

Department of Health (2001a). *Manual of Cancer Services Standards*. London: NHS Executive.

Department of Health (2001b). *Statistics on Smoking Cessation Services in the Health Action Zones in England, April 1999 to March 2000. Statistical Bulletin 2001/02* . London: Department of Health. Available online at: www.dh.gov.uk/assetRoot/04/02/24/22/04022422.pdf (accessed on 16 June 2006).

Department of Health (2000a). *The NHS Cancer Plan: A plan for investment, a plan for reform*. London: Department of Health.

Department of Health (2000b). *The NHS Plan: A plan for investment, a plan for reform*. London: The Stationery Office.

Department of Health (1999). *Saving Lives: Our healthier nation*. London: The Stationery Office.

Expert Advisory Group on Cancer to the Chief Medical Officers of England and Wales (1995). *A Policy Framework for Commissioning Cancer Services*. London: Department of Health.

Goodwin N (2004). 'Key lessons for network management in healthcare. Managers Making the Links'; IHM Annual Conference, SECC Glasgow. Available online at: http://ihm.atalink.co.uk/ articles/106 (accessed on 27 June 2006).

Grant J (2005). *Incentives for Reform in the NHS: An assessment of current incentives in the south-east London health economy*. London: King's Fund.

Hardcastle J, Chamberlain J, Robinson M, Moss S, Amar S, Balfour T, James P, Mangham C (1996). 'Randomised controlled trial of faecal-occult-blood screening for colorectal cancer'. *The Lancet*, vol 348, pp 1472–77.

Herbst R, Prager D, Hermann R, Fehrenbacher L, Johnson BE, Sandler A, Kris MG, Tran HT, Klein P, Li X, Ramies D, Johnson DH, Miller VA (2005). 'TRIBUTE: A Phase III trial of Erlotinib Hydrochloride (OSI-774) combined with Carboplatin and Paclitaxel chemotherapy in advanced non–small-cell lung cancer'. *Journal of Clinical Oncology*, vol 23, no 25, pp 5892–9.

Honore B, Lleras Muney A (2004). *Bounds in Competing Risks Models and the War on Cancer*. NBER Working Paper 10963. Cambridge MA: National Bureau of Economic Research, Inc.

House of Commons Committee of Public Accounts (2006). *The NHS Cancer Plan: A progress report*. Twentieth Report of Session 2005/06. London: The Stationery Office. Available online at: www.publications.parliament.uk/pa/cm200506/cmselect/cmpubacc/791/791.pdf (accessed on 16 June 2006).

House of Commons Hansard Debate (2005). Parliamentary questions on health. Available online at: www.publications.parliament.uk/pa/cm200506/cmhansrd/cmo50627/text/50627w43.htm (accessed on 27 June 2006).

House of Commons Science and Technology Committee (2002). *First Report, Cancer Research: A follow up*. HC444. London: The Stationery Office.

Kunkler I, James N, Maher J (2004). 'Cancer 2025: radiotherapy'. *Expert Review of Anticancer Therapy*, vol 4, 3s1, S37–41.

Leonard RCF, Smith IE, Coleman RE, Malpas JS, Nicolson M, Cassidy J, Jones A, McIllmurray MB, Stuart NSA, Woll J, Whitehouse JMA (1997). 'More money is needed to care for patients with cancer'. *British Medical Journal*, vol 315, pp 811–12.

McVie G, Schipper H, Sikora K (2004). 'Cancer 2025: Chemotherapy'. *Expert Review of Anticancer Therapy*, vol 4, 3s1, S43–50.

National Audit Office (2005a). *Tackling Cancer: Improving the patient journey*. London: The Stationery Office.

National Audit Office (2005b). *The NHS Cancer Plan: A progress report*. London: The Stationery Office.

National Audit Office (2004). *Tackling Cancer in England: Saving more lives*. London: National Audit Office.

NHS Breast Screening Programme (2002). *Breast Screening: A pocket guide*. London: NHS Cancer Screening Programme.

NHS Cancer Screening Programmes. 'Prostate Cancer Risk Management'. Available online at: www.cancerscreening.nhs.uk/prostate/index.html (accessed on 7 July 2006).

NHS End of Life Care Programme (2006). 'Welcome to End of Life Care Programme'. Available online at: http://eolc.cbcl.co.uk/eolc (accessed on 27 June 2006).

NHS Health and Social Care Information Centre (2006). *Breast Screening Programme, England: 2004/05*. Leeds: NHS Health and Social Care Information Centre. Available online at: www.ic.nhs.uk/pubs/brstscrnprogeng2005/FINALREPORT.pdf/file (accessed on 25 July 2006).

NHS Health and Social Care Information Centre (2005). *Cervical Screening Programme, England: 2004/05*. Leeds: NHS Health and Social Care Information Centre.

National Screening Committee UK (2005). 'National Screening Committee: Lung cancer screening'. Available online at: http://rms.nelh.nhs.uk/screening/viewResource.asp?uri=http://libraries.nelh.nhs.uk/common/resources/?id=61086 (accessed on 27 June 2006).

North London Cancer Network (2003). *North London Cancer Network Annual Report 2003*. London: North London Cancer Network.

Office for National Statistics (2006). 'National projections'. Downloaded from www.statistics.gov.uk/cci/nugget.asp?id=1352

Office for National Statistics (2005a). *Cancer Atlas of the United Kingdom and Ireland 1991–2000*. Basingstoke: Palgrave Macmillan.

Office for National Statistics (2005b). *Cancer Statistics Registrations: Registrations of cancer diagnosed in 2003, England*. London: ONS. Available online at: www.statistics.gov.uk/downloads/theme_health/MB1_34/MB1_34.pdf (accessed on 16 June 2006).

Office for National Statistics (2005c). 'Cancer Survival: Rates improved during 1996–2001'. Available online at: www.statistics.gov.uk/cci/nugget.asp?id=861 (accessed on 7 July 2006).

Peto J, Gilham C, Fletcher O, Matthews FE (2004). 'The cervical cancer epidemic that screening has prevented in the UK'. *The Lancet*; vol 364, pp 249–56.

Peto R, Darby S, Deo H, Silcocks P, Whitley E, Doll R (2000). 'Smoking, smoking cessation, and lung cancer in the UK since 1950: Combination of national statistics with two case-control studies'. *British Medical Journal,* vol 321, pp 323–29.

Peto R, Lopez AD, Boreham J, Thun M, Heath jnr C (1992). 'Mortality from tobacco in developed countries: Indirect estimation from national vital statistics'. *The Lancet*; vol 339, pp 1268–78.

Reid J (2003). *Localising the National Health Service: Gaining greater equity through localism and diversity*. London: The New Local Government Network.

Royal Society (2005). *Personalised medicines: Hopes and realities*. London: The Royal Society.

Scottish Executive Health Department (2001). *Cancer Scenarios: An aid to planning cancer services in Scotland in the next decade*. Edinburgh: The Scottish Executive.

Selby JV, Fiedman GD, Quesenberry CP, Weiss NS (1993). 'Effect of fecal occult blood testing on mortality from colorectal cancer: a case-control study'. *Annals of Internal Medicine,* vol 118, 1, pp 1–6.

Sikora K (2002). 'The impact of future technology care on cancer care'. *Clinical Medicine*, vol 2, 6, pp 560–68.

Stern R (1995). *Purchasing Small and Specialist Services*. Tonbridge: South East Institute of Public Health.

Summers E, Williams M (2006). *Re-audit of Radiotherapy Waiting Times 2005*. London: Royal College of Radiologists.

Swanton K, Frost M (2006). *Lightening the Load:Tackling overweight and obesity.* London: National Heart Forum. Available online at: www.heartforum.org.uk/Publications_NHFreports_ Overweightandobesitytool.aspx (accessed on 16 June 2006).

Tuyns AJ, Pequinot G, Jensen OM (1977). 'Le cancer de l'oesophage en Ille-et-Vilaine en fonction des niveaux de consommation d'alcool et de tabac. Des risques qui se multiplient'. *Bulletin du Cancer,* vol 64, 1, pp 45–60.

Wald N, Murphy P, Major P, Parkes C, Townsend J, Frost C (1995). 'UKCCCR multicentre randomised controlled trial of one and two view mammography in breast cancer screening'. *British Medical Journal,* vol 311, pp 1189–93.

Wells M, Harrow A, Donnan P, Davey P, Devereux S, Little G, McKenna E, Wood R, Chen R, Thompson A (2004). 'Patient, carer and health service outcomes of nurse-led early discharge after breast cancer surgery: A randomised controlled trial'. *British Journal of Cancer,* vol 91, pp 651–8.

World Health Organization (2003). *World Cancer Report.* Geneva: WHO.

World Health Organization (2002). *National Cancer Control Programmes: Policies and guidelines.* Geneva: WHO.